Flesh and Bones of
METABOLISM

Commissioning Editor: **Timothy Horne**
Development Editor: **Barbara Simmons**
Copy Editor: **Jane Ward**
Project Manager: **Frances Affleck**
Designer: **Jayne Jones**

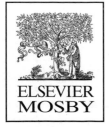

Flesh and Bones of
METABOLISM

Marek H Dominiczak MD FRCPath FRCP(Glas)

Consultant Chemical Pathologist
Clinical Biochemistry Service
NHS Greater Glasgow and Clyde
Gartnavel General Hospital, Glasgow, UK;
Honorary Senior Lecturer, University of Glasgow, UK;
Docent in Laboratory Medicine, University of Turku, Finland

Illustrations by Martin Woodward

ELSEVIER
MOSBY

Edinburgh   London   New York   Oxford   Philadelphia   St Louis   Sydney   Toronto   2007

**ELSEVIER
MOSBY**

First published 2007

ISBN-13: 978-0-7234-3368-2
ISBN-10: 0-7234-3368-2

British Library Cataloguing in Publication Data
A catalogue record for this book is available from the British Library

Library of Congress Cataloging in Publication Data
A catalog record for this book is available from the Library of Congress

Notice
Neither the Publisher nor the Author assume any responsibility for any loss or injury and/or damage to persons or property arising out of or related to any use of the material contained in this book. It is the responsibility of the treating practitioner, relying on independent expertise and knowledge of the patient, to determine the best treatment and method of application for the patient.
The Publisher

Printed in China

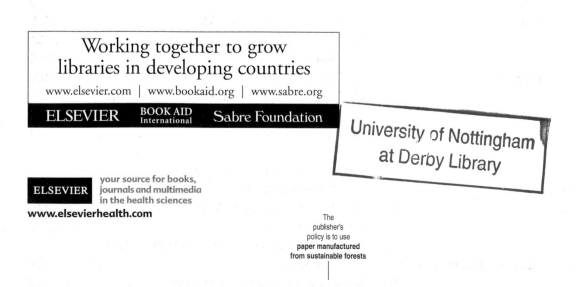

ELSEVIER your source for books, journals and multimedia in the health sciences

www.elsevierhealth.com

The publisher's policy is to use paper manufactured from sustainable forests

Contents

Preface

Biochemistry is the biological cousin of chemistry. In the generally overburdened medical curriculum, it is sometimes seen as something like a telephone directory of compounds and obscure formulae—and generally a largely irrelevant factual burden on the future medical mind. It should be neither; in fact, it is a fascinating subject, the knowledge of which can improve your clinical practice.

The understanding of biochemistry underpins molecular biology and it is of enormous value in understanding issues associated with nutrition. Knowledge of biochemistry does what science is supposed to do: makes one's decisions more rational and based on the understanding of underlying biological phenomena.

Unfortunately for the learner, biochemistry does have its own language specific to its needs: the chemical formulae that are graphical images of molecules. Take the structure of haem and try to describe it in detail: doing it without help of a chemical formula it would be a tedious task. Remembering formulae is largely unnecessary, but looking at them to facilitate understanding is useful. Similarly, a rudimentary knowledge of chemical bonding, and the basis for hydrophilicity (water-liking) and hydrophobicity (water-dislike), helps to imagine and understand biological phenomena such as the differences between the actions of steroid and polypeptide hormones.

The central premise of this book is that understanding biochemistry, and seeing the biochemical 'big picture' helps in learning clinical medicine. Therefore, the book omits much detail; it tries to give the reader an overall picture that can be filled in later with detail by reading larger textbooks. Another theme of this text is that the body, and metabolism, are closely linked to the environment, forming an open system that constantly communicates with the outside through gas exchange (oxygen and carbon dioxide) and nutrients and water intake and loss. In fact, many disorders have roots in the abnormalities of this communication, to mention only nutritional deficiencies, dehydration and overhydration and acid–base disorders.

During my clinical career, I have been involved in research on enzyme action, on insulin and glucagon, on diabetic complications and in clinical studies related to cardiovascular prevention and nutrition. All this was done while seeing thousands of patients. And, I have to say that I have always found biochemistry helpful in marshalling clinical thinking. This book, I hope, will convince some of you that this is indeed the case.

Marek H Dominiczak

Acknowledgements

Writing a single-author textbook, however small, is an exciting opportunity to present one's perspective on an impossibly wide subject. It also makes things easy for readers: they will know very clearly who to blame for mistakes and inadequate explanations.

During my career, I have always had to subject biochemistry —fascinating as it is—to verification by clinical practice and physician's judgments; some would call it introducing a subjective approach to hard science, others acknowledging science's uncertainties. Be that as it may, this book attempts to give a coherent, digestible picture of biochemistry to budding doctors, a picture with as many links as possible to problems they will deal with every day.

My thanks to all those I work with and learn from. I am particularly grateful to surgeons, residents and the Nutrition Team at Gartnavel General Hospital and the Western Infirmary in Glasgow; people who constantly, in their own words, keep me focused.

I am also much indebted to the team at Elsevier and particularly to Jane Ward, whose competence and knowledge of the subject made creation of this book a pleasure, and to my secretary, Jacky Gardiner, for her excellent, as usual, assistance.

Marek H Đominiczak

The big picture

Biochemistry is about chemical reactions in living organisms. Great progress has been made in our understanding of energy production, heredity and the chemical signals that regulate individual reactions and entire pathways—and make cells into a hugely complex, fantastically well-integrated system. Metabolism means 'all chemical reactions in the body'. Section one discusses the main concepts and interactions on a 'macro' scale. It presents an organism as an open system that constantly communicates with the environment through food intake, regulation of water balance, and gas exchange. It describes how such a system generates energy to survive. It looks at catalysts, which make complex reactions possible at neutral pH and relatively low temperature (enzymes) and at macro-regulators of metabolism (hormones). These concepts subsequently become underlying themes for defining anabolism and catabolism and the main chains (pathways) of reactions that occur in the body. Finally, we illustrate how energy metabolism relates to physiological conditions and to disease, and provide examples of how the seemingly theoretical science of biochemistry becomes very relevant to the art of being a good physician.

■ KEY CONCEPTS IN BIOCHEMISTRY

Metabolism encompasses all the chemical reactions that take place in a living organism. **Anabolic** reactions are those that lead to energy storage and to biosyntheses. **Catabolic** ones are those that lead to the release of energy and to degradation of compounds. Sequences of reactions leading to a particular endpoint are known as metabolic pathways.

To characterize a pathway, one first needs to know its place in the overall scheme and its purpose. Next, one needs to know its substrates and products, its regulatory mechanisms and its links with other pathways. However, it is the integrated operation of different pathways that creates the 'metabolic state' that a clinician observes in a hospital or an outpatient clinic. The greatest pitfall in trying to understand metabolism is to consider its fragments in isolation.

Biochemistry is chemistry applied to biology. Like chemistry, it has its own specific terms, and indeed a whole specific language: the chemical formulae. Familiarizing oneself with a handful of the most important concepts and trying to look at formulae as an informative alphabet of biochemistry requires a little effort at the start but pays off enormously further down the road. There is no escape from the fact that it is chemistry we are talking about here.

Therefore, in the big picture, we will first look at the basic concepts and at the main classes of compound (and chemical bond) that make up a cell. Then we will consider the most important metabolic pathways in an integrative manner and attempt to relate this knowledge to medical issues.

The organism as an open system

The organism is an open system; that is, it constantly communicates with the environment. Several different exchanges of chemicals take place. Most importantly, the intake of O_2 is required to allow oxidative energy-yielding reactions to take place.

Oxygen is taken in by the lungs and distributed to tissues throughout the cardiovascular system by a protein carrier, a metalloprotein, **haemoglobin**. This is linked to the excretion of CO_2 produced by the metabolism: in fact, the affinity of haemoglobin for O_2 changes as it circulates from the lungs (where higher pH favours O_2 binding) to the peripheral tissues (where lower pH favours O_2 dissociation). The O_2–CO_2 exchange is associated with buffering (i.e. the maintenance of a stable pH of the body fluids): CO_2 forms a part of the most efficient buffer system in the body, the **bicarbonate buffer**.

Water and electrolytes, such as sodium, chloride, potassium and magnesium, are required to maintain the internal environment. Their intake and excretion are regulated by two hormonal systems: vasopressin secreted by the posterior pituitary, which controls renal water excretion, and the renin–angiotensin–aldosterone system, which controls renal excretion of sodium and potassium ions.

Apart from O_2 and water, the organism requires a constant input of energy-containing metabolic fuels: the nutrients. The main classes of nutrient are **carbohydrates**, **proteins** and **lipids**.

Carbohydrates are the principal metabolic fuel, particularly in the short term. Their energy yield is 4 kcal/g. Importantly, glucose is the only fuel that the brain and erythrocytes can use in most situations; therefore, its constant supply is paramount. There is an emergency store of carbohydrates, **glycogen**, held in the liver and in muscle to provide fuel for short bursts of intense activity. However, carbohydrates also play a structural role in the body in addition to their role as a fuel, particularly in combination with lipids and proteins, as glycolipids and glycoproteins, respectively. Humans can synthesize all the carbohydrates they need.

Lipids, the second major class of nutrients, are the metabolic fuel with the highest caloric value, 9 kcal/g. They are stored principally in the adipose tissue as esters of fatty acids and glycerol (the **triacylglycerols**; also known as triglycerides) and are the principal fuel used when food is in short supply or when a prolonged energy expenditure is required. Two polyunsaturated fatty acids, linoleic and linolenic acid, cannot be synthesized in the body and have to be supplied with diet. Apart from being used as fuel, lipids, particularly the complex ones such as phospholipids and sphingolipids, play a key structural role in biological membranes. They also serve as signalling molecules in the hormonal systems. Most lipids, like glucose, are oxidized to CO_2 and water; the exception is the steroid nucleus (the structure of cholesterol), which cannot be metabolized and needs to be excreted with bile.

Proteins, the third major class of nutrients, are polymers of amino acids, organic acids that contain nitrogen. Proteins taken with food are digested and the constituent amino acids are used for synthesis of organism's native proteins. Out of the 20 amino acids, nine are essential—cannot be synthesized in the body—and need to be supplied with diet.

Proteins are responsible for most of the catalytic and regulatory activity within the organism. The principal catalytic molecules, **enzymes**, are proteins that bind substrates of chemical reactions and decrease the activation energy, so that reactions can proceed at body temperature and pH. Many proteins serve as regulatory compounds: **hormones, cytokines, growth factors** and **transcription factors**; some enzymes such as kinases and phosphatases are also regulatory as they control the function of other enzymes. The whole diverse system of proteins remains under genetic control and is encoded in the sequence of bases in the genome.

Although there is no specific 'storage' protein in the organism, the bulk muscle protein serves as a fuel reserve at times of need. If need arises (this happens, for instance, during prolonged fasting), the carbon skeletons of the amino acids are metabolized to the same intermediates as carbohydrates and used to produce energy. However, the nitrogen contained in the amino acids is toxic: during amino acid metabolism it is metabolized in the urea cycle, and its product, urea is excreted in urine. The difference between the nitrogen content of food and nitrogen excretion (the **nitrogen balance**) is an important marker of anabolic or catabolic state.

Coenzymes are low-molecular-weight substances that play an essential role in assisting enzymatic reactions but are not an integral part of the enzyme. **Vitamins**, a class of essential nutrients, serve as coenzymes in a range of chemical reactions. They may also serve as hormones (such as vitamin D). In some cases, they constitute prosthetic groups of enzymes (permanent parts of enzyme structure, as opposed to the reversibly bound coenzymes). Haem, for example, is the prosthetic group of haemoglobin, while nicotinae adenine dinucleotide (NADH) is a coenzyme in the conversion of pyruvate to lactate.

Finally, there is a nutritional requirement for metals such as iron, copper, manganese selenium and cobalt.

The vital interface in the process of nutrient assimilation is the gastrointestinal tract and associated organs, the pancreas and the liver. The efficiency of digestion and absorption is fundamental for nutrient uptake, and gastrointestinal disorders often lead to nutritional deficiencies and malnutrition.

An organism is an open system in that it constantly exchanges chemicals with the environment. Clinical examination and investigations assess the principal components of this system. This includes the examination of respiratory, cardiovascular and gastrointestinal systems, and renal function. Physicians routinely check O_2 delivery; test the haemoglobin concentration in blood; assess water balance, charting the fluid intake and loss; check electrolyte losses and their concentration in blood; and assesses the state of nutrition as well as the caloric balance and nitrogen balance.

Compartments within the open system

The entire organism and the individual cells contain many separate 'drawers' or compartments. The two major water and electrolyte compartments are the **intracellular** and the **extracellular fluid**. The intracellular fluid compartment is enclosed by cell membrane formed from a lipid bilayer. There is a free exchange of water between these two compartments, but the membrane is only selectively permeable to ions and larger molecules. To communicate with its environment, the membrane contains a host of **receptors** and **ion channels**. They, respectively, transduce metabolic signals carried by membrane-bound molecules, such as hormones, and facilitate selective uptake of substances into the cell and the maintenance of ionic and metabolite gradients. Some ion channels are receptors for signalling molecules. The intracellular fluid has a high potassium ions concentration (approximately 150 mmol/l) and is low in sodium ions. The reverse is true for the extracellular fluid. The sodium–potassium gradient maintained by the enzyme Na^+/K^+-ATPase is essential for the maintenance of cellular integrity and is fundamental for the propagation of nerve impulses along the nerve cell membranes. The concentration of calcium ions within different subcellular compartments (see below) is equally important: an increase in the cytoplasmic calcium ion concentration is a factor triggering muscle contraction and many secretory processes in the cell.

Interfaces similar to cell membrane (indeed formed by a similar lipid bilayer structure) exist between subcellular organelles: the cytoplasm, the mitochondria, nucleus, endoplasmic reticulum, lysosomes and peroxisomes (Fig. 1.1). The subcellular compartments separate reactions and pathways in a way that enables opposing processes, such as fatty acid synthesis and degradation,

to occur in the cell at the same time. Metabolites are transported between compartments by selective transport systems, such as dicarboxylate and tricarboxylate carriers in the inner mitochondrial membrane.

When key metabolites need to be transported between compartments, a number of so-called **metabolic shuttles** can be used in addition to transport systems; these shuttles are sequences of reactions that convert a non-transportable metabolite into a transportable one on one side of the barrier, thus bypassing the need for a specific transport system. For instance, the glycerol phosphate shuttle employs this principle to transport NADH to the mitochondria.

Figure 1.2 provides an overview of metabolism. Each of the elements shown in the figure is expanded upon in the following chapters.

Fig. 1.1 Cellular organelles.

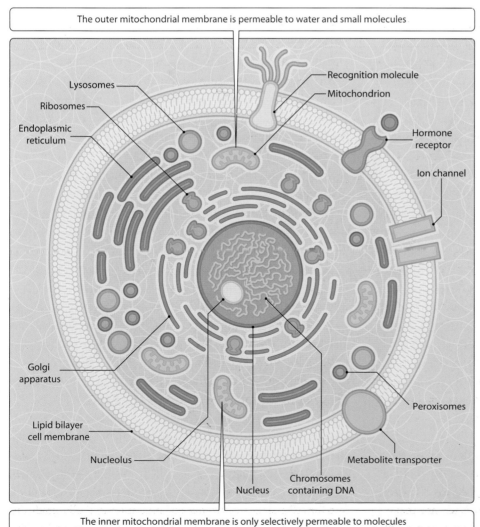

The outer mitochondrial membrane is permeable to water and small molecules

Recognition molecule
Mitochondrion
Lysosomes
Ribosomes
Endoplasmic reticulum
Hormone receptor
Ion channel
Golgi apparatus
Peroxisomes
Lipid bilayer cell membrane
Nucleolus
Metabolite transporter
Chromosomes containing DNA
Nucleus

The inner mitochondrial membrane is only selectively permeable to molecules

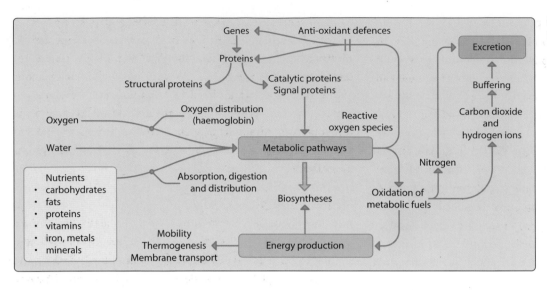

Fig. 1.2 The big picture of metabolism.

ENERGY

Reactions during which the degree of randomness (entropy) increases proceed spontaneously, with the release of energy (we call them exergonic). Reactions that decrease randomness need energy input in order to proceed (they are endergonic). Biological oxidations provide the energy for such reactions. A substantial part of the energy released during biological oxidations is trapped in the high-energy bonds of the nucleotide adenosine trisphosphate (ATP). ATP subsequently serves as an 'energy currency', because it is able to donate its energy to drive many biosynthetic reactions: it serves as a fundamental link between catabolism and anabolism.

Oxidation is essentially the extraction of electrons from the molecules of metabolic fuels and their transfer to molecular oxygen. This is a highly endergonic reaction, but in biological systems it proceeds stepwise and its energy is released in small portions. Electrons are extracted together with protons as energy substrates are oxidized. Next, these are transported to the mitochondrial respiratory chain by dedicated carriers: the nucleotides NADH and $FADH_2$. These nucleotides are reoxidized in the respiratory chain. The transport of electrons is associated with protons being pumped out of the mitochondrial matrix. The protons then return though an ion channel that is part of the enzyme ATP synthase; this movement of protons provides energy for ATP synthesis. ATP can also be produced outside the mitochondria, in substrate-level phosphorylations, but this is a minor contribution compared with the ATP yield of the respiratory chain.

Unfortunately, oxidations are not without potentially harmful effects. When the oxygen atom is not completely reduced (i.e. when it accepts just one electron instead of the two required for complete oxidation), oxygen forms highly reactive free radicals

(**reactive oxygen species** (ROS)) such as the superoxide or the hydroxy radical. They can chemically modify other compounds such as polyunsaturated fatty acids or proteins and impair their function. To prevent this, organisms possess enzymes that neutralize ROS: superoxide dismutase and catalase. The tripeptide glutathione also plays an important role in antioxidant defence, particularly in the erythrocytes. Excessive formation of ROS, or their inefficient removal, is known as **oxidative stress** and this contributes to the development of many chronic disorders such as diabetes mellitus, arthritis and atherosclerosis.

Biological catalysis and metabolic regulatory systems

Most chemical reactions in the body are catalysed by enzymes: proteins that possess substrate-binding active centres, binding to which decreases the energy required for a reaction to occur. Enzymes are often multisubunit structures, and occasionally form large, multifunctional complexes (such as pyruvate dehydrogenase or fatty acid synthetase). Importantly, they are subject to multiple controlling mechanisms. They can be regulated by allosteric effectors: low-molecular-weight ligands that alter the interaction between enzyme subunits, and thus substrate binding. Another powerful regulatory mechanism is phosphorylation and dephosphorylation of enzymes catalysed by enzymes known as kinases and phosphatases, respectively. The activity of these regulatory enzymes is controlled, in turn, by hormonal signals. Importantly, a hormone can, through signalling cascades, control kinases participating in several different metabolic pathways; this is how hormones coordinate different metabolic pathways. Rates of enzymatic reactions are often controlled by changes in the rate of enzyme synthesis (i.e. repression or activation of relevant gene).

The main pathway of ATP production

The backbone of energy metabolism is the transformation of glucose to CO_2 and water; this produces energy and conserves it in the storage molecules such as glycogen and lipids. One can consider **glycolysis**, the **Krebs cycle**, the **respiratory chain**, **glycogen synthesis** and **lipogenesis** as a large complex of anabolic reactions.

Glucose metabolism consists of glycolysis, the Krebs cycle the respiratory chain and the formation and degradation of glycogen. Both glycolysis and the Krebs cycle link to lipid deposition (lipogenesis). Other simple carbohydrates, such as fructose and galactose, link into glycolysis at its later stages and are then metabolized in this common pathway.

Glycolysis

Glycolysis is a cytoplasmic pathway that proceeds from glucose supplied either from plasma or from glycogen stored in liver and muscle. Importantly, glycolysis can operate both in aerobic and anaerobic conditions.

When O_2 is present, glycolysis yields pyruvate, which subsequently enters the mitochondrial Krebs cycle. In anaerobic conditions, however, pyruvate is reduced to lactate. Anaerobic glycolysis yields only a fraction of ATP produced during aerobic metabolism but is fundamental for, for instance, working muscle. Erythrocytes are entirely dependent on glycolysis because they do not have mitochondria.

Glycolysis has several branching points. It links to the **pentose phosphate pathway**, which generates the nucleotide NADPH for cytoplasmic biosyntheses and produces ribose phosphate for the synthesis of nucleotides and nucleic acids. Glucose metabolism yields the initial glycolytic metabolite glucose 6-phosphate; the final metabolite, pyruvate, can enter the Krebs cycle. Importantly, glycolysis also links to fat metabolism. One of the intermediates of glycolysis, dihydroxyacetone phosphate, is the precursor of glycerol, which, in turn, is essential for triacylglycerol synthesis (i.e. fat deposition). (Incidentally, this is how eating carbohydrates leads to weight gain.) Glycolysis is reciprocally regulated by insulin and glucagon, and the enzyme phosphofructokinase-1 is its main regulatory enzyme.

Krebs cycle

The Krebs cycle, also known as the tricarboxylic acid cycle, is the hub of all aerobic energy metabolism. In aerobic conditions, glycolysis is linked to the Krebs cycle through the transformation of pyruvate into acetyl-conezyme A (CoA), catalysed by pyruvate dehydrogenase. During the cycle, a 2-carbon molecule, acetyl-CoA, is converted to CO_2: the process yields large amounts of NADH and $FADH_2$, which enter the respiratory chain. The Krebs cycle enzymes are located in the mitochondria close to the respiratory chain.

The Krebs cycle supplies most of the electrons required to drive cellular ATP production. It also serves as a biochemical multijunction. It links to lipid metabolism through acetyl-CoA, and to amino acid metabolism through transamination reactions involving oxaloacetate and α-ketoglutarate. Krebs cycle intermediates may at the same time be both products of degradation of different compounds (catabolism) and substrates for biosyntheses (anabolism). We, therefore, say that the Krebs cycle is **amphibolic**.

Respiratory chain

The mitochondrial respiratory chain is the main site of ATP production in the cell during the oxidative phosphorylation. During this process, the electrons brought to the mitochondria by NADH or $FADH_2$ are transferred, through four multienzyme complexes in the inner mitochondrial membrane, to molecular O_2. This is combined with pumping the accompanying protons out of the mitochondrial matrix. The protons return through an ion channel in a fascinating molecular motor, the ATP-producing ATP synthase.

The pathways of energy storage

Energy supply needs to be constant but food supply is periodical. There are normally breaks of several hours between food ingestion, and the organism might need to survive much longer periods of fasting during illness or when food is in short supply. In fact, humans can survive up to approximately 180 days without food.

The additional complication is that in normal circumstances the brain can only use one fuel, glucose (during starvation it adapts partially to the use of ketone bodies). Therefore, irrespective of the food supply, a constant level of glucose is necessary for survival.

The ability to function without a continuous food supply results from the existence of energy storage pathways, and from the ability of the organism to convert its own structural proteins into glucose. Let us deal with the energy storage pathways first: they are glycogen synthesis (glycogenogenesis) and triacylglycerol synthesis (lipogenesis).

Glycogen

Glycogen is the polymer of glucose that is stored in liver and in muscle. It is a large highly branched molecule packed in a way that leaves many 'loose ends' accessible to degradative enzymes. The main difference between the two storage sites of glycogen (liver and muscle) is the way of glucose release: while glucose derived from liver glycogen can be released to the blood through the action of glucose-6-phosphatase, muscle is only able to use its released glucose for its own needs.

Glycogen synthesis is stimulated by insulin and takes place in the fed state. The key enzymes in glycogen synthesis are glycogen synthase, which adds glucose residues linearly, and the branching enzyme, which constructs chemical bonds at different positions, creating a non-linear structure. Glycogen is synthesized from glucose after glucose has been phosphorylated within the cell to glucose 6-phosphate and then glucose 1-phosphate.

Lipogenesis: synthesis of fatty acids and triacylglycerols

The energy-rich lipids synthesized for energy storage are the hydrophobic long-chain fatty acids. They are stored in the adipose tissue as esters with glycerol (**triacylglycerols** or triglycerides).

The fatty acids are synthesized in the liver and, in particular, adipose tissue whenever there is abundance of carbohydrates in food. Their immediate precursor is the acetyl-CoA derived from aerobic glycolysis. The rate-limiting step is the enzyme acetyl-CoA carboxylase, which is regulated by acetyl-CoA itself and also by citrate, insulin, glucagon and epinephrine (adrenaline). Fatty acids are subsequently esterified to triacylglycerols. In fat cells, the source of glycerol is the glycolytic intermediate dihydroxyacetone phosphate.

Fats in the diet can also be converted into storage triacylglycerols. After digestion, they are transferred from the intestine to adipose (and other) tissues in lipoprotein particles known as **chylomicrons**. Chylomicron triacylglycerols are hydrolysed and fatty acids taken up by cells for storage.

Energy supply during fasting

When the food supply ceases, the entire energy metabolism changes direction within few hours. The change involves shutting down the anabolic pathways, glycogenogenesis and lipogenesis, and activating glycogen degradation (**glycogenolysis**), **lipolysis** and another pathway essential for ensuring the long-term continuity of glucose supply, **gluconeogenesis**. This dramatic reconfiguration of metabolism is directed by the reciprocal changes in the secretion of two hormones: **insulin** and **glucagon**. Fasting suppresses insulin secretion and stimulates the secretion of glucagon (the insulin-to-glucagon ratio in the circulation decreases). Epinephrine, released from the adrenal cortex, also plays an important role in this. These pathways are discussed in turn.

Release of glucose from glycogen

The hallmark of glycogen release is its immediacy. Release is controlled by a cascade-like intracellular signalling system, which responds to glucagon and epinephrine.

Glucagon and epinephrine bind to their membrane receptors. This stimulates conformational changes in small membrane-associated proteins called **G-proteins** and results in the stimulation of an enzyme **adenylyl cyclase** producing a cyclic nucleotide, cyclic adenosine monophosphate (**cAMP**). This, in turn, stimulates protein kinase A, which is able to phosphorylate other kinases, thus disseminating the hormonal signal. The outcome is the phosphorylation, and associated change in activity, of several key enzymes participating in glycogenolysis/glycogenogenesis, glycolysis and lipolysis/lipogenesis.

Glycogen phosphorylase is activated and, acting in sequence with the debranching enzyme, it degrades glycogen to glucose 1-phosphate, which is then converted to glucose 6-phosphate. The glucose 6-phosphate enters glycolysis or (in the liver) is converted to glucose and released into the bloodstream. Note that glycogen release is also controlled by neural signals and plays a key role in the 'fight and flight' reaction.

Lipolysis and the oxidative metabolism of fatty acids (beta-oxidation)

In contrast to the immediate supply of energy from glycogen, lipolysis is a pathway geared to long-term supply of energy. It is closely linked with the oxidation of fatty acid molecules to acetyl-CoA, which then enters the Krebs cycle.

Lipolysis is the degradation of triacylglycerols to glycerol and fatty acids. It is controlled by **hormone-sensitive lipase**, an enzyme that is one of the regulatory targets of glucagon and epinephrine (both stimulate the lipase).

Fatty acid oxidation requires the transport of the fatty acids to the mitochondria; this is accomplished by a membrane shuttle involving the alcohol carnitine. Fatty acids are degraded into 2-carbon fragments yielding large amounts of NADH and acetyl-CoA.

Further metabolism of acetyl-CoA in the Krebs cycle depends on the availability of the cycle intermediate oxaloacetate. Acetyl-CoA condenses with oxaloacetate, forming citrate. When there is not enough oxaloacetate available, the excess acetyl-CoA is directed to ketogenesis: a short pathway resulting in the production of acetoacetate, β-hydroxybutyrate and acetone (the **ketone bodies**). Ketogenesis is a sort of metabolic stop-gap solution. The ketone bodies can be recycled to acetyl-CoA and used as fuel later on. However, ketone bodies are acids, and so if they are present in large amounts they cause acidosis (this happens in diabetes mellitus and is known as diabetic ketoacidosis).

Gluconeogenesis

Gluconeogenesis is an essential catabolic pathway activated by fasting. It is the pathway of glucose production from non-carbohydrate sources. It supplies glucose to blood during fasting and during prolonged exercise. Gluconeogenesis takes place in the liver and, to a lesser extent, in the kidneys. Muscle is incapable of gluconeogenesis because it does not possess glucose-6-phosphatase, the enzyme that releases glucose from cells.

The main gluconeogenic substrates are the amino acid **alanine**, the lipid **glycerol** and the glycolytic metabolite **lactate** (the last is important in recovery from anaerobic exercise). Because alanine can be synthesized from other amino acids by transamination, it provides a portal for directing muscle amino acids into energy metabolism. Importantly then, gluconeogenesis provides a way to use muscle protein to produce energy. Gluconeogenesis is not a reverse of glycolysis: its key regulatory enzymes are phosphoenolpyruvate carboxykinase (PEPCK) and fructose-1-6-bisphosphatase. Similarly to glycogenolysis, and lipolysis, its principal regulators are glucagon and epinephrine. Importantly, the key metabolite of gluconeogenesis is oxaloacetate: it is the depletion of oxaloacetate during active gluconeogenesis that redirects acetyl-CoA towards ketone body production.

Providing glucose inhibits gluconeogenesis and in consequence spares muscle protein. This protein-sparing action of glucose is one of the principles underlying nutrition during illness.

A closer look at amino acid metabolism

As mentioned above, amino acids can be used as substrates to produce glucose. To serve this purpose, most of them are first converted to glutamate or alanine. The fundamental reaction that enables the conversion of amino acids is **transamination**: here an amino acid reacts with the keto acid pyruvate or a metabolite of the Krebs cycle; the transfer of the amino group takes place, forming a 'new' pair of amino and keto acids.

In fact, amino acids are metabolized to several energy substrates: those that yield glycolytic metabolites (in particular pyruvate) are known as **glucogenic**. Amino acids that produce acetyl-CoA or acetoacetate are known as **ketogenic**. Some amino acids can be both gluco- and ketogenic.

However, amino acids contain nitrogen, which is toxic to tissues. The entry portal for nitrogen removal is the amino acid glutamate and its derivative glutamine. Glutamate can release nitrogen by oxidative deamination catalysed by glutamate dehydrogenase (other amino acids can be converted to glutamate by transamination). The nitrogen released as the ammonium ion reacts with bicarbonate, forming carbamoyl phosphate, which enters the cycle of **urea synthesis** in the liver. Urea serves as the vehicle for urinary nitrogen excretion. In fact, measurement of urinary nitrogen excretion has been used to assess nitrogen metabolism. The nitrogen balance is the difference between nitrogen intake and its urinary output. A positive nitrogen balance indicates the anabolic state, and a negative balance indicates a catabolic state.

Medical relevance of the pathways of energy metabolism

The postprandial state and the fed state
Organisms alternate between the fasting state and the fed state. This is highly relevant to many diagnostic procedures. Fasting is regarded as the metabolic reference state, and performing laboratory tests during fasting is particularly important for the diagnosis of diabetes and lipid disorders.

Exercise
Muscular exercise is a good illustration of the sequential use of different energy sources by the organism. The exercising muscle relies on ATP and its regeneration from another high-energy compound, **creatine phosphate**, for short bursts of activity. Exercise lasting several minutes requires the activation of glycogenolysis by epinephrine and glucagon. Intensive, short-term exercise relies on anaerobic glycolysis from glycogen. The energy for longer-lasting (endurance) exercise is provided by fatty acid oxidation, with parallel contribution by gluconeogenesis.

Stress and injury are the catabolic states most frequently observed by a clinician
Stress and injury induce the 'fight and flight' reaction. Importantly, the reaction of organisms to stress is controlled by both the nervous and the endocrine systems. It is initiated in the hypothalamus and involves both pituitary (adrenocorticotrophic hormone) and effector endocrine glands (adrenal cortex, medulla and pancreas). The activation of the sympathetic nervous system is fundamental in this. Metabolically, the stress response can be regarded as a comprehensive anti-insulin response. Epinephrine and glucagon activate glycogenolysis. Insulin concentration decreases, sparing glucose for the brain use. Chronic stress involves activation of gluconeogenesis and lipolysis. Importantly, stress and injury are associated with a degree of immunosuppression, and also with a cytokine-mediated inflammatory response. This underlies the increased susceptibility to infections that is seen in acutely ill and injured patients.

Diabetes mellitus
Diabetes mellitus is a common metabolic disease that involves primarily carbohydrate and lipid metabolism. Type 1 diabetes (previously known as juvenile diabetes or insulin-dependent diabetes (IDDM)) is caused by insulin deficiency, and type 2 diabetes (previously known as non-insulin-dependent diabetes (NIDDM)) by a combination of insulin resistance and deficient secretion. In diabetes, the effect of anti-insulin hormones prevails, leading to active gluconeogenesis (i.e. glucose production by the liver) and ongoing fatty acid oxidation.

Diabetes is characterized by hyperglycaemia, leading to long-term tissue damage, and by the risk of acute decompensation, known as diabetic ketoacidosis. A common complication of diabetes, particularly of insulin-treated diabetes, is hypoglycaemia. Both diabetic ketoacidosis and severe hypoglycaemia are medical emergencies.

In diabetes, chronic hyperglycaemia and disordered lipid metabolism lead to long-term complications such as eye (retinopathy), kidney (nephropathy) and peripheral nerve (neuropathy) damage. An important role in this is played by oxidative stress induced by hyperglycaemia. Diabetes is also associated with macroangiopathy, leading to atherosclerosis and cardiovascular disease.

A major risk factor for type 2 diabetes is obesity, where the common denominator seems to be the insulin resistance caused predominantly by defective insulin signalling. Importantly, weight reduction decreases the chance of development of diabetes in obese individuals.

Atherosclerosis

Atherosclerosis is a common disease of large arteries. It involves endothelial dysfunction, lipid (particularly low density lipoproteins (LDL)) deposition in the arterial wall, the proliferation and intimal migration of the arterial smooth muscle cells, and an inflammatory reaction that involves macrophages and T lymphocytes and change the structure of the arterial wall. Atherosclerosis leads to coronary heart disease, stroke and peripheral vascular disease, and it is a leading cause of mortality worldwide.

■ THE BIOSYNTHETIC MACHINERY

Synthetic pathways related to amino acid metabolism

In parallel to the energy-supplying pathways, there is a wide range of biosynthetic reactions operative at any time. Many of those are linked to the metabolism of amino acids.

Apart from the nine amino acids that need to be supplied in the diet, the amino acids can be synthesized from either glycolytic or Krebs cycle metabolites such as pyruvate, oxaloacetate or phosphoenolpyruvate. Apart from serving as building blocks for protein synthesis, amino acids are substrates for the synthesis of many specialized molecules such as purine and pyrimidine nucleotides, the hormone thyroxine, the O_2-carrier haem and the neurotransmitters epinephrine and norepinephrine.

Importantly, inborn errors leading to deficiencies of enzymes involved in the synthesis and degradation of amino acids cause many rare metabolic diseases observed mostly in newborns and children. The most important of those is phenylketonuria, a defect in the metabolism of phenylalanine. Untreated, it causes mental retardation. This might be prevented by a phenylalanine-free diet. Large neonatal screening programmes have been set up for the early detection of phenylketonuria.

Porphyrins

Porphyrins are intermediates in the synthetic pathway of haem. They are synthesized from the Krebs cycle metabolite succinyl-CoA and the amino acid glycine. Haem contains an iron atom that is essential for O_2 binding. Defects in haem synthesis lead to rare diseases called porphyrias, characterized by hepatotoxicity and/or photosensitivity. Individual defects can be characterized by measuring different porphyrin metabolites (particularly porphobilinogen) in blood and urine.

Haem is metabolized to bilirubin. The measurements of bilirubin concentration in blood, together with the activities of liver enzymes, are extensively used in the differential diagnosis of liver disease.

Purines, pyrimidines and nucleic acids

Purines and pyrimidines are nitrogen-containing bases that, in combination with ribose phosphate, form nucleotides.

Nucleotides are involved in energy entrapment (ATP and GTP), the activation of synthetic substrates (UTP) and electron and proton transfer (NAD^+ and FAD). They are also constituents of nucleic acids, deoxyribonucleic acid (DNA) and ribonucleic acid (RNA). The synthesis of purines involves the amino acids glutamine and glycine, tetrahydrofolate, a derivative of the vitamin folic acid, and CO_2, supplied as bicarbonate. Pyrimidine synthesis involves the amino acids aspartate and glutamine, and bicarbonate.

Purines are metabolized to uric acid. Excess uric acid production or decreased excretion lead to gout.

Synthetic pathways related to lipid synthesis

Cholesterol

Cholesterol is a steroid that is an essential component of cell membranes, increasing their fluidity. It is synthesized from acetyl-CoA and its synthesis involves 5-carbon isoprene units. Cholesterol is a substrate for the synthesis of steroid hormones and vitamin D. It cannot be metabolized in the body and it is excreted with bile. It is transported in blood in lipoprotein particles, and cholesterol-rich remnant particles and LDL are atherogenic. The rate-limiting step in cholesterol synthesis is the enzyme hydroxymethylglutaryl (HMG)-CoA reductase. Intracellular cholesterol concentration controls the activity of HMG-CoA reductase, HMG-CoA synthetase and also the expression of the membrane LDL receptor.

Nucleic acids and protein synthesis

The nucleic acid DNA contains the set of genes (the **genome**) that code for all the proteins expressed throughout the life of an organism (the **proteome**). The sets of expressed genes are tissue specific, and the gene expression profile changes with age. The replication of DNA provides the basis for heredity (the transmission of genetic information from one generation to another). Gene expression is subject to multiple controls that involve nutrients and metabolic intermediates.

DNA and RNA

The nucleic acids RNA and DNA are polymers of purine and pyrimidine nucleotides. They have a double-helix structure maintained by hydrogen bonds between the complementary bases (adenine–thymine and guanine–cytosine; with uracil instead of cytosine in RNA). RNA participates in the transcription of the genes (messenger (mRNA)) and in their translation into the sequence of amino acid chains (transfer (tRNA)). RNA also, together with proteins, forms the infrastructure of the ribosomes (rRNA).

Protein synthesis

Protein synthesis takes place on the ribosomes where the coding sequence of the mRNA is translated into the amino acid sequence of a protein chain. The synthesis requires aminoacyl-tRNA, the RNA polymerase enzyme, and a host of protein initiation, elongation and termination factors. During protein synthesis, the ribosome advances along the mRNA chain and the newly synthesized protein is alternatively bound to two active centres on the ribosome. Specific codons signal the initiation and termination of polypeptide chain synthesis.

Protein synthesis is an energy-consuming process and increases in the anabolic state.

Gene expression

Gene transcription is controlled by promoter sequences upstream of the mRNA transcription start point. The controlling factors (**transcription factors**) are proteins possessing specific DNA-binding domains and these bind to DNA-response elements in the promoter region. Some genes are activated or suppressed by a combination of transcription factors. Transcription factor activation can be triggered by hormones, cytokines (growth factors) and some metabolic intermediates such as polyunsaturated fatty acids.

■ GENOMICS AND PROTEOMICS

The progress achieved in genomics and proteomics adds an entire new dimension to biochemistry as we know it. The elucidation of relationships between genes and disease promises to lead to more-precise diagnosis and genetic counselling, and also to new ways of treatment (gene therapy). The new discipline of **pharmacogenomics** looks into the possibilities of customizing drug treatments to the genetic make-up of an individual. Analogously, nutritional genomics should allow predictions to be made regarding the effects of diet, and dietary recommendations could be customized to individual metabolic responses. Proteomics, the large-scale monitoring of protein expression in health and disease, promises to give us a better picture of both metabolic changes and regulatory mechanisms in health and disease.

Biochemistry is constantly changing and offering new tools to those who look after patients. If anything, this is an important argument for learning it and keeping track of its development.

High return facts

Key concepts in biochemistry

1 Metabolism is the sum of all the chemical reactions that take place in the living organism. Anabolic reactions are those that lead to energy storage and to biosyntheses. Catabolic ones are those that lead to the release of energy and to degradation of compounds.

2 The strongest chemical bonds are the covalent bonds where two atoms (such as carbon atoms) share electron orbitals. However, biomolecules are also held together by an array of weaker interactions including hydrogen bonding, ionic and hydrophobic interactions and van der Waal's forces. These weak interactions are particularly important in the assembly of cellular membranes, proteins and nucleic acids.

3 Energy transfer underpins all metabolism. Energy released during biological oxidations is trapped in high-energy bonds, particularly the γ-phosphodiester bond of the nucleotide adenosine trisphosphate (ATP). ATP is subsequently able to transfer its energy to drive a host of biosynthetic reactions: it thus serves as a vital link between catabolism and anabolism.

4 Biological oxidations are essentially the extraction of electrons from substances used as metabolic fuels. Electrons are often extracted together with protons. They are then transported to the respiratory chain by the reduced proton/electron carriers such as NADH and $FADH_2$, which are reoxidized in the respiratory chain with the electrons being transferred, in several stages, to molecular O_2.

5 Hydrogen ions (protons) are produced during biological oxidations. The concentration of hydrogen ions (expressed as pH) determines the degree of ionization of molecules. The stability of body pH is maintained by buffer systems that minimize the pH changes on addition of an acid or a base. The main body buffers are the bicarbonate system, haemoglobin and phosphate. The components of the bicarbonate buffer are linked to atmospheric CO_2, which increases its buffering capacity.

6 Water provides the environment for most chemical reactions. Maintaining the water balance is fundamental for survival. Water intake is controlled by thirst and water loss by the hypothalamic hormone vasopressin, which acts on the collecting ducts of the kidney. Sodium and potassium balance is regulated by the renin–angiotensin–aldosterone system. Water movement between cell compartments is driven by the osmotic pressure.

7 Enzymes are catalytic protein molecules. They bind substrates in their active centres and create a transition state, a state of higher energy that allows a reaction to proceed. Enzymes are subject to several controls, such as positive and negative feedback effects exerted by metabolic intermediates. Allosteric interactions (where an effector binds to an area other than the active site and alters the conformation of the enzyme) and phosphorylation/dephosphorylation are particularly important regulatory mechanisms.

8 Vitamins perform the role of coenzymes and serve as enzyme prosthetic groups; some, such as vitamin A or vitamin D, have hormone-like actions. They are conventionally classified into fat soluble (membrane crossing) and water soluble. Vitamins A, D, E and K are fat soluble.

9 The water-soluble vitamins cannot be stored in the body for long and so diet-induced deficiencies occur more easily than for the fat-soluble vitamins. Water-soluble vitamins include vitamins of the B complex, vitamin C and folate. As they act as coenzymes in a wide range of reactions, deficiencies can cause non-specific symptoms.

10 Hormones are macro-regulators of metabolism. The organization of the endocrine system is hierarchical. Multilevel endocrine axes include the hypothalamus (secreting releasing hormones), the pituitary (secreting trophic hormones) and the effector glands such as the adrenal, thyroid, ovaries or testes.

11 Peptide and protein hormones do not cross cell membranes and exert their effect through membrane receptors, by triggering complex intracellular signalling cascades. Steroid hormones are hydrophobic and cross lipid bilayer membranes. They bind to their cytoplasmic receptors, which are ligand-activated transcription factors. The activated hormone–receptor complexes migrate to the nucleus where they bind to DNA-response elements, regulating gene expression.

12 Steroid hormones are derived from cholesterol and are synthesized in the adrenal cortex and gonads. Mineralocorticoids control electrolyte and fluid balance. The glucocorticoids contribute to the control of energy metabolism particularly during stress. The sex steroids control growth, sexual maturity and fertility.

13 Derivatives of the amino acid phenylalanine (and its metabolite tyrosine) serve as neurotransmitters, mediators of nerve impulses at neuronal synapses. Epinephrine, secreted by the adrenal medulla, and norepinephrine, secreted at neuronal synapses, are key mediators of the sympathetic nervous system. Acetylcholine is lipid-derived transmitter in the parasympathetic nervous system.

14 Signalling systems are sequences of reactions that translate information contained in hormone molecules into metabolic effects. Many polypeptide hormones act through a pathway comprising a membrane receptor, a G-protein, adenylyl cyclase and protein kinase A. They also signal through a pathway involving the hydrolysis of membrane phospholipids by phospholipase, generating diacylglycerols and inositol phosphates. The cytoplasmic concentration of calcium ions is also fundamental for hormone signalling.

15 Oxygen delivery to tissues is accomplished by the cardiorespiratory system and by distribution of O_2 through the blood, using the protein O_2 carrier haemoglobin. The affinity of haemoglobin for O_2 (and for CO_2, which it also transports) is regulated by the surrounding pH (the Bohr effect) and by the glycolytic metabolite 2,3-bisphosphoglycerate.

The key compounds

16 Amino acids are organic acids containing nitrogen in the form of the amino groups. They are zwitterionic molecules, acting as acids or bases depending on the pH. Formation of a peptide bond between a carboxyl group of one amino acid and an amino group of the other provides the backbone of protein molecules.

17 The side chains of amino acids determine the diversity of proteins, and the properties of the side chains determine protein folding. Amino acids with non-polar and aliphatic side chains will cluster in the centre of a molecule, avoiding water. Polar uncharged side chains or positively charged groups contribute to protein structure by forming non-covalent bonds. Rigid amino acids, such as proline, and amino acids contain sulphur, which can form disulphide bridges, giving rigidity to protein structure.

18 The sequence of amino acids in proteins is encoded in deoxyribonucleic acid (DNA); therefore the set of proteins synthesized in the body (the proteome) reflects the information contained in the genome. The primary structure of protein (the sequence of amino acids covalently joined by peptide bonds) determines the secondary (folding of the chain of amino acids into spiral helices, flat sheets or wavy sheets, held together by weak interactions) and the tertiary (organization of the helices and sheets in space) structures. Interactions between protein subunits determine quarternary structure.

19 Carbohydrates include simple sugars (monosaccharides and disaccharides) and complex ones (polysaccharides) such as starch or glycogen. Carbohydrates (principally glucose) are used as a metabolic fuel, and ribose is an essential component of nucleotides and nucleic acids. Carbohydrates also form complex molecules with lipids and proteins (glycolipids and glycoproteins, respectively).

20 Fatty acids provide high-calorie metabolic fuel, and their esters with glycerol (triacylglycerols, also known as triglycerides) are the main storage fuel in the adipose tissue. Phospholipids are essential components of biological membranes, and both phospholipids and fatty acids serve as signalling molecules.

Energy metabolism

21 Digestion converts nutrients into their elemental components, which are absorbed into the plasma from the gastrointestinal tract. Carbohydrates are digested to monosaccharides, lipids to mono- and diacylglycerols, and proteins to their component amino acids.

22 Lipoproteins are lipidated protein molecules. They are classified as chylomicrons, high density lipoproteins (HDL), very low density lipoproteins (VLDL), remnant particles and low density lipoproteins (LDL).

23 Lipids (both those absorbed from the intestine and those synthesized de novo in the liver) are transported between organs as components of lipoprotein particles. A system of removal of cholesterol from cells by high density lipoproteins (HDL) is known as reverse cholesterol transport.

24 Glycolysis is the core cytoplasmic pathway of glucose (and energy) metabolism. It can proceed from either glucose or glycogen. It operates both in aerobic and anaerobic conditions. In the presence of O_2, it yields pyruvate, which enters the Krebs cycle. In anaerobic conditions, it yields lactate.

25 Glycolysis has both energy-consuming and energy-yielding steps. The net yield is 2ATP from each molecule of glucose.

26 The Krebs cycle, also known as the tricarboxylic acid cycle, is the hub of aerobic metabolism, integrating carbohydrate, lipid and protein metabolism and creating a common gateway to the mitochondrial respiratory chain. It links to glycolysis through the pyruvate dehydrogenase reaction, which yields acetyl-CoA from pyruvate.

27 The Krebs cycle converts the 2-carbon molecule of acetyl-CoA to CO_2: the process yields NADH and $FADH_2$, which subsequently enter the respiratory chain. The cycle is also a hub where many metabolic pathways converge.

28 The mitochondrial respiratory chain is the main site of ATP production in the cell. It accepts electron carriers NADH and $FADH_2$ for reoxidation. This takes place in a stepwise manner: it involves four enzymatic complexes, ending with the transfer of electrons to molecular O_2. The passage of electrons along the respiratory chain is associated with pumping of protons out of the mitochondrial matrix. The protons return through an ion channel, which is a part of the enzyme ATP synthase. The process linking electron transfer to ATP synthesis is known as oxidative phosphorylation.

29 Metabolic shuttles are sequences of reactions that allow the transfer of molecules across a membrane that is normally impermeable to them without the need for a direct transport mechanism. Neither NADH nor acetyl-CoA can cross the inner mitochondrial membrane; metabolic shuttle mechanisms enable the transfer of NADH into the mitochondria where it enters the respiratory chain, and the movement of acetyl-CoA out of the mitochondria to participate in cytoplasmic biosynthetic reactions.

30 The pentose phosphate pathway is a branch of glycolysis. In this pathway, glucose 6-phosphate is oxidized yielding NADPH for use in the cytoplasmic lipogenesis and the regeneration of reduced glutathione; the pathway also generates ribose 5-phosphate for the synthesis of nucleotides.

31 Glycogen serves as an energy store. It provides an emergency fuel for the brain if supply in the bloodstream is inadequate. In muscle, it is essential for bursts of activity associated with the 'fight and flight' reaction.

32 A hormone-responsive signalling system enables the instant use of glycogen. Glycogen release is controlled by both metabolic and neural signals. The principal hormones that control glycogenolysis are glucagon and epinephrine. Insulin promotes glycogen synthesis.

33 Gluconeogenesis is the pathway of glucose production from non-carbohydrate sources. It supplies glucose during prolonged periods of fasting and during exercise. The main gluconeogenic substrates are the amino acid alanine, the lipid glycerol and the glycolytic metabolite lactate.

34 As gluconeogenesis and glycolysis occur in the same cell compartment and utilize a number of common enzymes, strict control mechanisms are required to ensure glucose is utilized and formed to physiological requirements. The three key enzymes are controlled by small molecules acting as allosteric effectors, by covalent changes to the enzymes and by changes in the concentrations of the enzymes. Hormonal regulation provides integration with other tissues and pathways.

35 Lipolysis is the degradation of triacylglycerols to glycerol and fatty acids. It is controlled by hormone-sensitive lipase, an enzyme regulated by glucagon and epinephrine. The fatty acids are then degraded into 2-carbon fragments, yielding NADH and acetyl-CoA, by a series of oxidative reactions known as beta-oxidation.

36 Ketogenesis occurs when there is an excess of acetyl-CoA derived from the beta-oxidation of fatty acids. It generates the so-called ketone bodies: acetoacetate, β-hydroxybutyrate and acetone. Ketone bodies can be used as a fuel by muscle, and also by the brain during periods of starvation. Excessive ketogenesis is the hallmark of diabetic ketoacidosis.

37 Fatty acids are synthesized from acetyl-CoA. The rate-limiting step is acetyl-CoA carboxylase, which is regulated by acetyl-CoA itself and also by citrate, insulin, glucagon, and epinephrine. Fatty acids can then be incorporated into triacylglycerols, the storage form of neutral fat, by reaction with glycerol phosphate. Lipogenesis is stimulated by insulin.

38 Pyruvate, oxaloacetate and acetyl-CoA are the three key metabolites linking different pathways in fuel metabolism. Pyruvate links glycolysis with the Krebs cycle, participates in anaerobic glycolysis (where it is converted to lactate) and can be transaminated to alanine. Oxaloacetate is a key Krebs cycle metabolite that condenses with acetyl-CoA to form citrate. It is also a key substrate for gluconeogenesis. Acetyl-CoA is probably the most universal of the three. It can be generated from pyruvate or from the fatty acid oxidation. If unable to enter the Krebs cycle, it enters ketogenesis. It also serves as a substrate for many biosynthetic reactions including fatty acid and cholesterol synthesis.

39 There is no storage of amino acids in the body and so they are replenished from dietary protein and any excess is excreted. Glutamate and glutamine are formed by transamination reactions from α-ketoglutarate and other amino acids.

40 Amino acid breakdown gives rise to carbon skeletons and nitrogen. The carbon skeletons are metabolized to energy substrates. Amino acids that can be metabolized to glycolytic or Krebs cycle intermediates are known as glucogenic, and those that yield acetyl-CoA or acetoacetate are known as ketogenic. Some amino acids are both gluco- and ketogenic. Nitrogen from amino acids is eliminated through the urea cycle after being incorporated into carbamoyl phosphate. The urea is excreted in urine.

The key biosynthetic pathways

41 Cholesterol is synthesized from the acetyl-CoA. The rate-limiting enzyme in cholesterol synthesis is hydroxymethylglutaryl (HMG)-CoA reductase. Cholesterol is also a substrate for the synthesis of steroid hormones and vitamin D. It cannot be metabolized in the body and is excreted in the bile (both in the native form and as bile acids).

42 Porphyrins are intermediates in the pathway of haem synthesis. They are synthesized from the Krebs cycle metabolite succinyl-CoA and the amino acid glycine. Haem contains an iron atom essential for O_2 binding. Haem is metabolized to bilirubin.

43 Amino acids are synthesized either from glycolytic or Krebs cycle metabolites such as pyruvate, oxaloacetate or phosphoenolpyruvate or from (in case of the essential amino acid histidine) a carbohydrate, ribose phosphate. The 11 non-essential amino acids can be synthesized in the human. Nine amino acids are essential for human metabolism but cannot be synthesized in the body; these are made in bacteria or plants and are acquired with diet.

44 Purines and pyrimidines are nitrogen-containing bases that, in combination with ribose phosphate, form nucleotides involved in energy transfer (ATP and GTP), activation of biosynthetic substrates (UTP in the synthesis of glycogen) and proton transfer (NAD^+ and FAD). They are key constituents of nucleic acids: deoxyribonucleic acid (DNA) and ribonucleic acid (RNA).

45 The nucleic acids RNA and DNA are polymers of purine and pyrimidine nucleotides. They can form double-helical structures maintained by hydrogen bonds between the complementary bases (adenine–thymine and guanine–cytosine in DNA; uracil instead of cytosine in RNA). The set of genes in DNA (the genome) contain the information for the amino acid sequences of all the proteins that the organism can synthesize.

46 DNA is replicated by unwinding the helix and synthesizing a complementary strand along its length. It is transcribed into mRNA and non-coding sequences are removed. The genes in mRNA are then translated into the sequence of amino acid chains (transfer RNA (tRNA)). Ribosomal RNA and proteins make up the protein-synthesizing organelle, the ribosome.

47 Protein synthesis takes place on the ribosomes, where the coding sequence of the mRNA is translated into the amino acid sequence of a polypeptide chain.

48 The synthesis requires activated amino acids in the form of aminoacyl-tRNA, the enzyme RNA polymerase and an array of protein initiation, elongation and termination factors. Protein synthesis requires energy in the form of ATP and GTP.

49 Gene transcription is controlled by promoter sequences upstream of the mRNA transcription start point. The controlling factors (transcription factors) are proteins possessing specific DNA-binding domains that bind to DNA-response elements in the promoter region. A single transcription factor may affect the expression of several genes, or the expression of a single gene can be regulated by two or more transcription factors.

Application of biochemistry to medicine

50 Nutrition provides a vital link between an organism and the environment. The principal classes of nutrient are carbohydrates (yielding 4 kcal/g), fats (9 kcal/g) and proteins (4 kcal/g). Alcohol yields 7 kcal/g. Other nutrients are vitamins, electrolytes and trace metals. Water intake is essential for survival.

51 The organism alternates between fed and fasted state. The fed state is promoted by insulin and is an anabolic condition with main pathways directed towards energy accumulation. Fasting induces a decrease in the insulin-to-glucagon ratio in plasma. As a consequence, anabolic pathways are suppressed. During fasting, the plasma glucose concentration is initially maintained by glycogenolysis. With time, stimulation of gluconeogenesis takes place, together with the stimulation of lipolysis and of beta-oxidation of the fatty acids. Excess lipolysis may lead to ketogenesis. An increase in the concentration of ketone bodies in blood is the hallmark of a prolonged fasting and starvation.

52 Insulin and glucagon are key hormones regulating energy metabolism. Both are produced in the pancreas and have actions at multiple sites. Insulin resistance in target tissues impairs glucose metabolism and is associated with type 2 diabetes and obesity.

53 Insulin and glucagon are controlled by the concentration of metabolic fuels, primarily glucose. Insulin and glucagon exert coordinated, and opposite, action on fuel metabolism pathways: glycolysis, gluconeogenesis, glycogen synthesis and breakdown, and lipolysis and lipogenesis. While insulin is the only hypoglycaemic/anabolic hormone, glucagon action is assisted by other hormones with anti-insulin action, notably epinephrine and cortisol.

54 During exercise, muscle relies on ATP and its regeneration from creatine phosphate for short bursts of activity. Glycolysis from glycogen becomes the main source of energy during short-term exercise. Longer exercise requires energy from fat oxidation and glucose production through gluconeogenesis.

55 Stress and injury induce a catabolic state and the 'fight and flight' reaction. Reaction to stress is controlled by both nervous and endocrine systems. It is initiated in the hypothalamus and involves both the pituitary (adrenocorticotrophic hormone) and effector endocrine glands (particularly adrenal cortex, adrenal medulla and pancreas). Activation of the sympathetic nervous system is fundamental to the stress response.

56 Obesity is a common problem and is associated with a considerable burden of disease, including diabetes, cardiovascular disease, gallstones and bone and joint disorders. Obesity is associated with changes in secretion of hormones (adipokines such as leptin or adiponectin) from adipose tissue and, in particular, with tissue resistance to insulin.

57 Diabetes mellitus is a common disorder, primarily of carbohydrate and lipid metabolism, caused by either insulin lack (type 1 diabetes) or a combination of insulin resistance and defective insulin secretion (type 2 diabetes). In diabetes, the effect of anti-insulin hormones

prevails: the characteristic feature is hyperglycaemia and glucosuria caused by decreased tissue glucose uptake and active gluconeogenesis (i.e. glucose production by the liver). There is increased lipolysis and fatty acid oxidation. In decompensated diabetes, the excess acetyl-CoA enters ketogenesis, and this may lead to diabetic ketoacidosis.

58 The long-term complications of diabetes, microangiopathy (retinopathy and nephropathy), macroangiopathy (atherosclerosis) and neuropathy (demonstrating both microangiopathic and metabolic/osmotic components), are caused by the toxicity of glucose and lipid metabolites. Oxidant stress seems to play a key role in their development. Maintaining good control of plasma glucose concentration (glycaemic control) has been shown to prevent or delay development of complications.

59 Starvation is associated with a catabolic response, which includes beta-oxidation of fatty acids, ketosis and gluconeogenesis (leading to muscle wasting). Malnutrition is characterized primarily by weight loss (marasmus), when structural proteins are preserved, or by ensuing oedema (kwashiorkor) when they are not. Apart from areas of famine, malnutrition may be a problem in hospitalized patients and in elderly populations.

60 Atherosclerosis is a disease of large arteries. It involves endothelial dysfunction, lipid (particularly low density lipoproteins) deposition in the arterial wall, proliferation and intimal migration of the arterial smooth muscle cells, and an inflammatory reaction involving macrophages and T lymphocytes. The arterial wall loses its ordered structure and there is narrowing of the arterial lumen by atherosclerotic plaque. The principal atherosclerosis-related diseases are coronary heart disease, stroke and peripheral vascular disease.

61 Many aspects of biochemistry are translated into practice in the clinical laboratories, which perform a wide range of tests on blood, urine, cerebrospinal fluid or surgical drainage samples (peritoneal fluid or joint aspirates). Timing of samples and appropriate collection procedures are important for obtaining clinically meaningful results.

62 Biochemistry-informed approach to a patient involves the integration of clinical signs and symptoms with information on O_2 delivery, anabolic or catabolic state, water and electrolyte balance, acid–base status and nutrition. Assessment of the metabolic status of a patient needs to be a part of daily clinical practice for every physician and surgeon. This is the approach that this book hopes to promote.

Fleshed out

Section three contains chapters as double page spreads, each expanding the specific high return fact presented in Section two. It aims to facilitate deeper understanding of the underlying concept. The nature of compounds and chemical bonds, energy production, and enzymes and hormones as catalysts and regulators of reactions and pathways are discussed in more detail as are the mechanisms of intracellular signal generation and the nature of these signals: topics that underlie much of the current thinking in therapeutic interventions. Then, the individual pathways of energy metabolism, and key biosynthetic processes are described. The final part expands on the application of biochemistry to medicine and discusses the biochemical basis of the most common physiological states, such as fasting and feeding, exercise and stress. It also illustrates the relevance of these states to the development of disease, with examples of conditions that are at the focus of today's public health concerns: obesity, diabetes mellitus and atherosclerosis. Finally, some pointers are given on how to integrate this knowledge into clinical practice through the use of the biochemistry tests available in hospital laboratories.

1. Metabolism

Questions
- Which reactions, anabolic or catabolic, are usually associated with oxidation?
- Name two multienzyme complexes
- What is the role of compartmentalization of pathways in the regulation of metabolism?

Metabolism encompasses all chemical reactions in the body, including those generating energy, maintaining body temperature, supporting biosyntheses, maintaining ion balances, eliminating toxic products and so on. **Anabolic** reactions are geared to fuel storage, biosynthesis and growth and **catabolic** reactions to energy release and substance degradation. Energy metabolism is an extremely slow and tightly controlled combustion (oxidation). In physics terms, it means extraction of electrons from fuel molecules and their transfer to molecular oxygen.

Metabolic pathways

Metabolic pathways are sequences of reactions. Physical proximity of the reacting substrates is important: some pathways are catalysed by **multienzyme complexes**, large macromolecules comprising several enzymatic activities such as the pyruvate dehydrogenase complex. Pathways may operate across cellular compartments separated by biological membranes. Because membrane transport is highly selective, compartments are linked by membrane-embedded transport systems (e.g. the dicarboxylate carrier); some pathways contain bypass systems (**metabolic shuttles**) that link sections (e.g. the carninine shuttle in fatty acid oxidation).

Regulation of pathways

Pathways are subject to many regulatory mechanisms (Fig. 3.1.1). Regulation at the entire pathway level tends to be exerted by hormones, working through influence on protein (enzyme) synthesis or enzyme activity. The latter is commonly achieved by enzyme phosphorylation. Hormones such as insulin and glucagon employ phosphorylation and dephosphorylation of enzymes to shift the entire metabolism towards anabolism (insulin) or catabolism (glucagon).

The availability of substrates can also be regulatory; for example, acetyl-CoA from beta-oxidation of fatty acids enters the Krebs cycle if there is sufficient oxaloacetate and otherwise is directed into ketogenesis. Individual metabolites can alter the activity of multimeric enzymes in pathways other than their primary one by changing the shape of the enzyme through binding to it at a site distant from the active site (**allostery**); for instance, citrate, a Krebs cycle metabolite, inhibits the glycolytic enzyme phosphofructokinase-1.

A common regulatory mechanism is feedback inhibition, where the final product inhibits a key upstream (rate-limiting) reaction (e.g. haem inhibits D-alanine synthetase). Forward activation occurs when a metabolite affects downstream reactions in a pathway (e.g. fructose 1,6-bisphosphate activates pyruvate dehydrogenase).

Finally, cellular compartments separate degradative from biosynthetic pathways (e.g. lipolysis from lipogenesis) and maintain separate pools of metabolites (e.g. mitochondrial and cytoplasmic acetyl-CoA) (Fig. 3.1.2). Figure 3.1.3 is an overview of linkage of pathways by common metabolites and usage of the same coenzymes.

CATABOLIC STATE IN INFECTIONS

A 62-year-old man was admitted with increasing breathlessness, which had been developing for 3 days. He had fever of 38.5°C and had not eaten for 36 hours. Pneumonia was diagnosed and sputum cultures revealed a staphylococcal infection. Infection like this is a classic example of a catabolic state, the main pointers here being the period of fasting and fever. One should also look for recent weight loss.

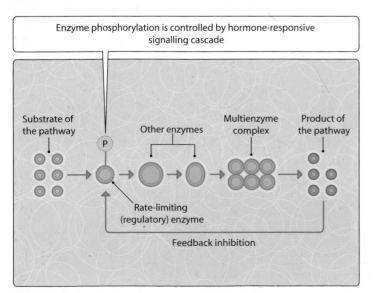

Fig. 3.1.1 Metabolic pathways and their regulation.

Fig. 3.1.2 The compartmentalization of metabolic pathways.

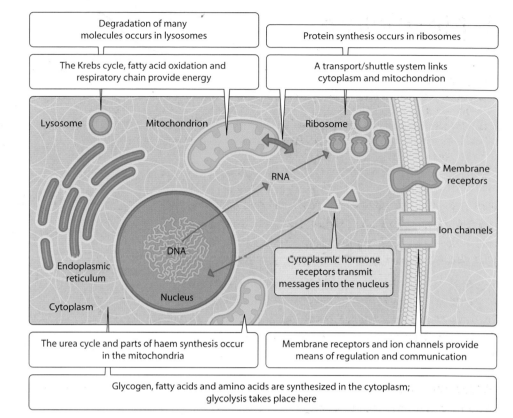

Degradation of many molecules occurs in lysosomes

Protein synthesis occurs in ribosomes

The Krebs cycle, fatty acid oxidation and respiratory chain provide energy

A transport/shuttle system links cytoplasm and mitochondrion

Lysosome

Mitochondrion

Ribosome

RNA

Membrane receptors

Ion channels

Endoplasmic reticulum

DNA

Cytoplasmic hormone receptors transmit messages into the nucleus

Nucleus

Cytoplasm

The urea cycle and parts of haem synthesis occur in the mitochondria

Membrane receptors and ion channels provide means of regulation and communication

Glycogen, fatty acids and amino acids are synthesized in the cytoplasm; glycolysis takes place here

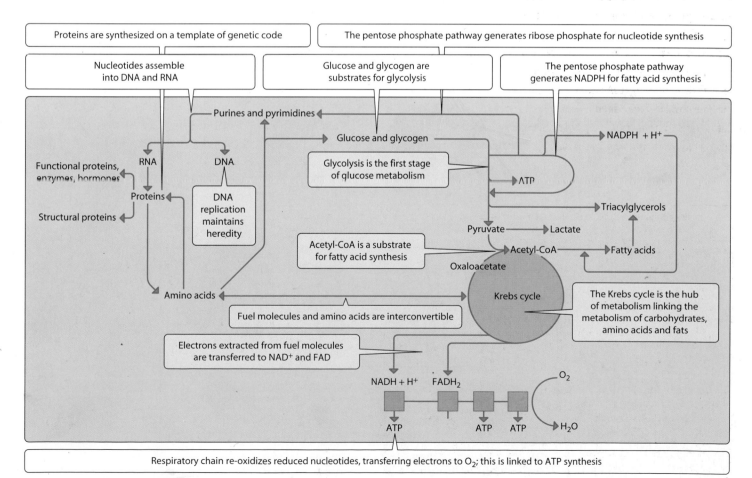

Proteins are synthesized on a template of genetic code

The pentose phosphate pathway generates ribose phosphate for nucleotide synthesis

Nucleotides assemble into DNA and RNA

Glucose and glycogen are substrates for glycolysis

The pentose phosphate pathway generates NADPH for fatty acid synthesis

Purines and pyrimidines

Glucose and glycogen

$NADPH + H^+$

Functional proteins, enzymes, hormones

RNA

DNA

Glycolysis is the first stage of glucose metabolism

ATP

Proteins

DNA replication maintains heredity

Triacylglycerols

Structural proteins

Pyruvate

Lactate

Acetyl-CoA is a substrate for fatty acid synthesis

Acetyl-CoA

Fatty acids

Oxaloacetate

Amino acids

Krebs cycle

The Krebs cycle is the hub of metabolism linking the metabolism of carbohydrates, amino acids and fats

Fuel molecules and amino acids are interconvertible

Electrons extracted from fuel molecules are transferred to NAD$^+$ and FAD

$NADH + H^+$

$FADH_2$

O_2

ATP

ATP   ATP

H_2O

Respiratory chain re-oxidizes reduced nucleotides, transferring electrons to O$_2$; this is linked to ATP synthesis

Fig. 3.1.3 Cellular metabolism: an overview.

2. Biologically important chemical bonds

Questions
- Which types of bond are responsible for protein folding?
- Give examples of hydrogen bonds
- How are hydrophobic and hydrophilic residues orientated in the biological membranes?

Molecules are held together by chemical bonds. These bonds differ in strength. The strong ones are the covalent bonds such as C–C or C–H. However, there are several weaker interactions that are very important in biology. These are:

- hydrogen bonds
- ionic interactions
- van der Waals forces
- hydrophobic interactions.

The chemical bonds present in a living organism include the 'backbone' of covalently bound molecules (Fig. 3.2.1), but complex structures such as folded protein chains, polysaccharides or biological membranes depend on these weak interactions.

Non-covalent bonds

Hydrogen bonds

Electronegative atoms such as O or N attract hydrogen. Hydrogen bonds also form between dipoles of water (Fig. 3.2.2) and between amino acid residues of proteins (the oxygen atoms of carbonyl groups and the hydrogen atoms of the amino groups; Fig. 3.2.3) when these groups are accessible on protein surface. When protein chains are tightly packed inside molecules so that water is not accessible, hydrogen bonds may form within the same molecule. This type of bonding plays a major role in stabilizing the conformation of proteins, nucleic acids and polysaccharides. Hydrogen bonds are particularly important in maintaining the double-helical structure of the DNA (Fig. 3.2.4).

Ionic interactions

Ionic interactions are based on the attraction of oppositely charged groups between residues in the same molecule, for example an ionized carboxyl group (COO^-) and a protonated amino group (NH_3^+).

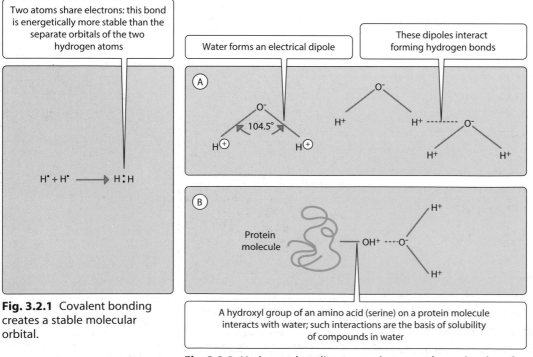

Fig. 3.2.1 Covalent bonding creates a stable molecular orbital.

Fig. 3.2.2 Hydrogen bonding occurs between the molecules of water and between other molecules and water; this is the basis for solubility of compounds.

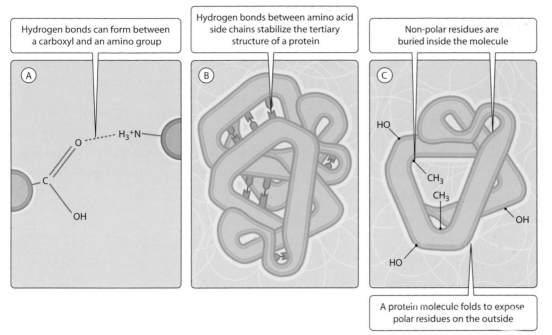

Fig. 3.2.3 Hydrogen bonds stabilize the structure of proteins.

Van der Waals forces

Van der Waals forces are weak interactions that act at short distances: in close proximity molecules start to repel each other.

Hydrophobic interactions

Hydrophobic residues do not form hydrogen bonds with water. Water repels them and they tend to cluster away from the water interface. Such molecules locate within the core of proteins or lipoproteins and, in particular, within biological membranes (Fig. 3.2.5) Hydrophobic interactions, similarly to hydrogen bonds, stabilize molecules.

Collective effect of weak interactions

Note that different weak interactions can occur in the same molecule. Although individually these interactions are weak compared with the covalent bond, their collective strength is substantial. Also, because these interactions are based on diverse principles, it is relatively difficult to break all the bonds at the same time. One, therefore, can view most protein molecules and biological membranes as complex constructs held together by a constantly changing array of weak interactions.

Hydrophobic, hydrophilic and amphipathic molecules

Molecules that possess both polar and non-polar residues are called **amphipathic**: they have both hydrophilic and hydrophobic domains. Such molecules (for instance phospholipids) orient themselves at the water interface so that the polar heads face water and the non-polar residues locate away from it. This is the basis for the formation of phospholipid bilayers, the principal structure of biological membranes. In membranes, the polar heads of phospholipids interact with water, while non-polar acyl residues are held away from water. Some vitamins, sterols and proteins are also amphipathic. This concept is also relevant to the folding of protein molecules; when a protein chain folds, hydrophobic amino acids pack inside in a way that minimizes contact with water (this is the energetically optimal conformation) and the polar residues locate on the outside.

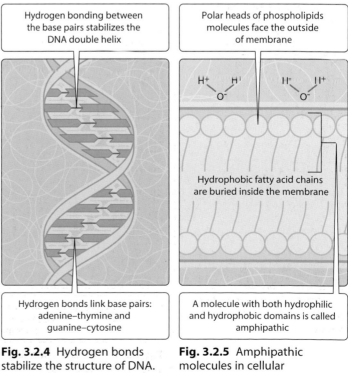

Fig. 3.2.4 Hydrogen bonds stabilize the structure of DNA.

Fig. 3.2.5 Amphipathic molecules in cellular membranes.

3. Energy

Questions

- Which reaction will progress spontaneously: the one linked to a positive or a negative change of free energy?
- What is the role of phosphate groups in energy transfer?
- Which are the major compounds involved in electron transfer?

Energy transfer underpins all metabolism. Considerations of metabolic energy are based on the two laws of thermodynamics:

- the first law states that the amount of energy in a system is constant
- the second law states that the entropy of systems tends to increase, and that any system progresses towards increased disorder (randomness).

The change in entropy is difficult to measure. Instead, we measure the **change in the free energy** (G) (Fig. 3.3.1) of reactants.

$$dG = G_{initial} - G_{final}$$

Negative change in free energy (less free energy at the completion of reaction) means that the reaction releases energy (is exergonic) and therefore can progress spontaneously. A positive change in free energy means that the reaction requires an input of energy to proceed (is endergonic).

The change of free energy is closely related to the equilibrium constant of a reaction (Fig. 3.3.1). The equilibrium constant (K_{eq}') of a reaction such as

$$A + B \rightleftharpoons C + D$$

is essentially a ratio between the concentration of reaction products and reaction substrates:

$$K_{eq}' = [C][D]/[A][B]$$

If in the reaction

$$A + B \rightleftharpoons C + D$$

the equilibrium constant is greater than 1, it means that at equilibrium there are more products than substrates (i.e. the reaction proceeds spontaneously). If the equilibrium constant is less than 1, it means that at equilibrium there will be still more substrates than products (therefore the reaction does not proceed spontaneously).

Energy transfer

Biochemical reactions proceed in energetically favourable direction (Fig. 3.3.2). Endergonic (energy-releasing) reactions proceed spontaneously, and exergonic ones require input of energy (activation energy). Energy is preserved in biochemical systems as the energy of chemical bonds. It can be transferred between different compounds. Energy transfer is most often associated

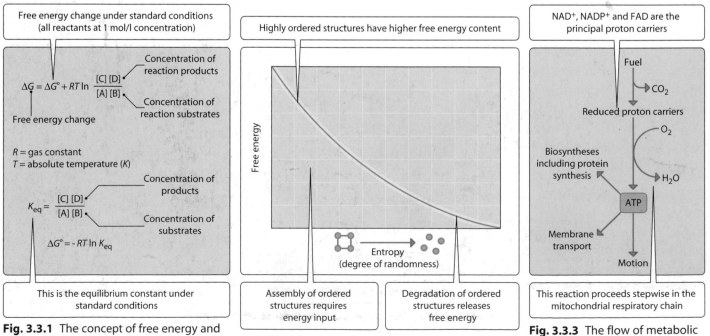

Free energy change under standard conditions (all reactants at 1 mol/l concentration)

$$\Delta G = \Delta G° + RT \ln \frac{[C][D]}{[A][B]}$$

Free energy change

Concentration of reaction products

Concentration of reaction substrates

R = gas constant
T = absolute temperature (K)

$$K_{eq} = \frac{[C][D]}{[A][B]}$$

Concentration of products

Concentration of substrates

$$\Delta G° = -RT \ln K_{eq}$$

This is the equilibrium constant under standard conditions

Fig. 3.3.1 The concept of free energy and the equilibrium constant.

Highly ordered structures have higher free energy content

Free energy

Entropy (degree of randomness)

Assembly of ordered structures requires energy input

Degradation of ordered structures releases free energy

Fig. 3.3.2 Entropy.

NAD^+, $NADP^+$ and FAD are the principal proton carriers

Fuel

CO_2

Reduced proton carriers

O_2

Biosyntheses including protein synthesis

H_2O

ATP

Membrane transport

Motion

This reaction proceeds stepwise in the mitochondrial respiratory chain

Fig. 3.3.3 The flow of metabolic energy.

with the transfer of phosphate groups: the common currency of energy in the cell is a nucleotide containing high-energy phosphate bonds, **adenosine triphosphate** (ATP) (Fig. 3.3.3). ATP is produced during exergonic reactions and the energy it 'traps' can subsequently be used to drive endergonic ones. The production of ATP is central to sustaining life. The most important sources of the ATP are the oxidation reactions in the mitochondrial respiratory chain. Reactions that produce high-energy compounds outside the respiratory chain are known as **substrate-level phosphorylations**.

Reactions may be driven by the hydrolysis of an energy-rich compound such as ATP or GTP (guanosine trisphosphate) or by lowering the energy of activation. Many reactions (such as carboxylation or the attachments of amino acids to transfer RNA) are driven by hydrolysis of pyrophosphate (written as PP_i).

The principal high-energy compounds

Adenosine triphosphate (ATP). ATP is a molecule consisting of a nucleoside, adenine, and a sugar, D-ribose (Fig. 3.3.4). Adenine and ribose are joined by the glycosidic bond. Ribose is highly phosphorylated: it contains three phosphate residues joined by anhydride bond. The two terminal phosphate groups (β and γ) are linked by high-energy bonds.

Creatine phosphate. Creatine phosphate is a high-energy compound essential for providing instantly available energy for short bursts of muscular exercise. It is able to convert ADP to ATP in a reaction

$$\text{creatine phosphate} + \text{ADP} \rightleftharpoons \text{ATP} + \text{creatine}$$

Compounds that mediate electron (and proton) transfer

Three nucleotides (Fig. 3.3.5) are involved in electron transfer:

- nicotinamide adenine dinucleotide (NAD^+)
- nicotinamide adenine dinucleotide phosphate ($NADP^+$)
- flavin adenine dinucleotide (FAD) (also flavin adenine mononucleotide FMN).

NAD^+ is a derivative of the vitamin nicotinamide and FAD is a derivative of riboflavin.

NAD^+ serves as a coenzyme in many catabolic and anabolic reactions. $NADP^+$ participates primarily in biosyntheses. FAD and FMN form prosthetic groups (an integral part of the enzyme molecule) rather than coenzymes.

The structure of NAD includes the adenine nucleotide and N-ribosyl nicotinamide linked by a pyrophosphate bond. $NADP^+$ has a phosphate group at position 2 of the adenosine ribose.

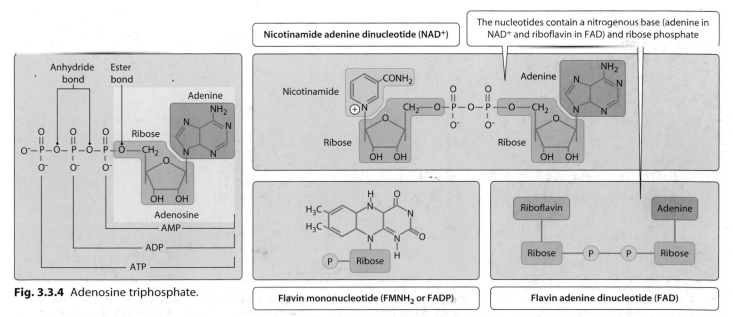

Fig. 3.3.4 Adenosine triphosphate.

Fig. 3.3.5 The compounds that mediate electron transfer.

4. Biological oxidations

Questions
- How is the process of oxidation explained in terms of electron exchange?
- Would an oxidizing agent donate or extract electrons from a molecule?
- What is oxidative stress?

Oxidation reactions underpin cellular energy production. However, in some circumstances they may be harmful.

Oxidation and reduction

Oxidation is essentially extraction of electrons. Therefore, an oxidizing agent is the electron-extracting agent. Oxidation is always combined with reduction (i.e. electron donation). Therefore, a reducing agent is an atom or a compound that supplies electrons (Fig. 3.4.1).

Electrons are transferred together with protons (hydrogen ions). This is why dehydrogenation is equivalent to oxidation (because electrons are lost together with protons), and hydrogenation is a reduction (electrons and protons are gained).

The tendency to donate electrons is known as **redox** (oxidation–reduction) **potential**. It can be quantified by comparing the electrical potential generated by a given pair of compounds with that of the hydrogen electrode as a reference. The more negative the reduction potential, the greater the tendency to donate electrons.

The most important oxidizing (electron-extracting) agent is O_2. Oxygen extracts electrons because its molecule does not possess a complete octet of electrons in one shell and it has two unshared electrons. When O_2 reacts with two hydrogen atoms, it extracts two electrons, forming water.

$$2H + \tfrac{1}{2}O_2 \rightleftharpoons H_2O$$

This is a highly exergonic reaction that underpins all biological oxidations: in biological systems it proceeds stepwise (see respiratory chain).

Oxygen free radicals: the reactive oxygen species

Oxygen needs to be activated to participate in metabolism; this can be accomplished by metal ions such as iron or copper. Metals donate a single electron to oxygen, yielding a partly oxidized oxygen atom, the **superoxide anion**, which is a highly reactive free radical (Fig. 3.4.2). The sources of oxygen free radicals (also known as reactive oxygen species (ROS)), apart

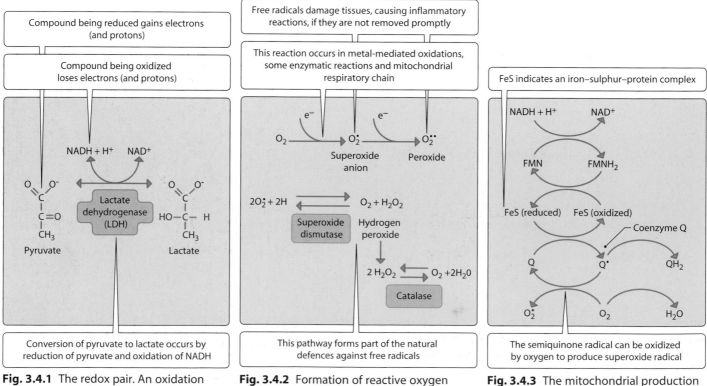

Fig. 3.4.1 The redox pair. An oxidation reaction is always combined with a reduction.

Fig. 3.4.2 Formation of reactive oxygen species (ROS) and their elimination by catalase and superoxide dismutase.

Fig. 3.4.3 The mitochondrial production of reactive oxygen species.

from metal-catalysed oxidations, are some enzymatic reactions (such as xanthine oxidase in the metabolism of purines) and, importantly, the reactions taking place in the respiratory chain (Fig. 3.4.3).

Oxygen, or nitrogen, free radicals are damaging to tissues, so conditions in which they are generated should be minimized. Such damage stimulates inflammatory reactions. **Oxidative stress** is a condition where the generation of free radicals exceeds the body's capacity to eliminate them (Fig. 3.4.4). Oxidative stress-associated tissue damage may be one of the causes of ageing, diabetic complications and atherosclerosis. The body possesses a system to guard against oxidant species: it includes the enzymes superoxide dismutase and catalase (Fig. 3.4.2), and the small peptide glutathione (Fig. 3.4.5).

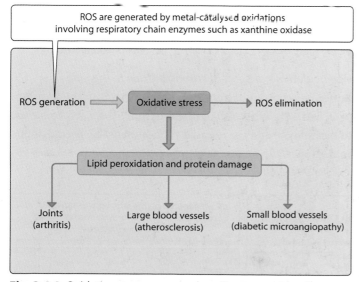

Fig. 3.4.4 Oxidative stress occurs when the generation of reactive oxygen species (ROS) exceeds the body's capacity for their elimination.

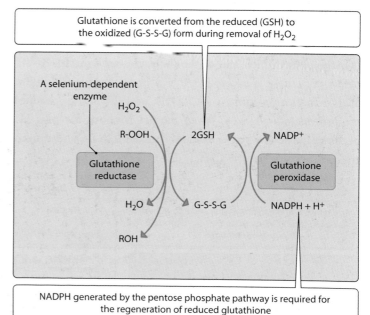

Fig. 3.4.5 Glutathione is a part of antioxidant defences.

7. Enzymes

Questions
- What is the function of a ligase?
- Will a competitive inhibition result in the change of enzyme K_m?
- What is an example of allosteric regulation?

Enzymes are proteins that serve as biological catalysts. They provide the activation energy for reactions (Fig. 3.7.1). Substrates bind to the active centre of an enzyme, which spatially fits the substrate.

Enzyme structure
Enzymes may comprise several subunits, and such subunits may interact to construct the active centre. Multienzyme complexes; facilitate interactions between substrates and products. Enzymes catalysing the same reaction may fulfil different functions in different cell compartments, for example, mitochondrial carbamoyl phosphate transcarbamoylase (CPS I) participates in the urea cycle, whereas cytosolic CPS II participates in porphyrin synthesis.

Enzyme kinetics
Enzyme binds a substrate, which is converted into a product and released.

$$E + S \rightleftharpoons ES \rightleftharpoons E + P$$

Enzyme activity is characterized by the Michaelis constant (K_m), which is the dissociation constant (K_d) of the enzyme–substrate complex (the lower the K_d the tighter the binding). The Michaelis constant is the substrate concentration at which the enzyme achieves 50% of its maximum velocity (Fig. 3.7.2).

Units of enzyme activity
Enzymes can be measured as protein concentration or enzyme activity: 1 kat is the catalytic activity that will raise the rate of a reaction by 1 mol/s. The international unit (IU) is the amount of enzyme that converts substrate at 1 mmol/min. The specific activity of an enzyme is expressed in IU/mg protein.

Types of enzyme
The classification developed by the Enzyme Commission (EC) assigns a four digit EC number to describe class and subclass.

1. Oxidoreductases: catalyse oxidation–reduction reactions
2. Transferases: catalyse group transfer, e.g. aminotransferases
3. Hydrolases: catalysc hydrolysis reactions
4. Lyases: catalyse addition of groups to double bonds or creation of a double bond by group removal
5. Isomerases: catalyse transfer of groups within a molecule
6. Ligases: catalyse condensation reactions.

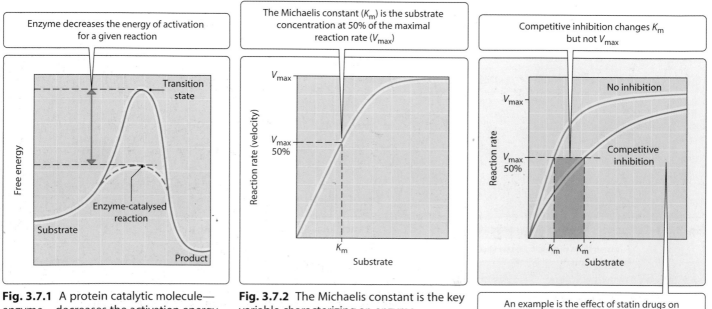

Fig. 3.7.1 A protein catalytic molecule—enzyme—decreases the activation energy of a reaction.

Fig. 3.7.2 The Michaelis constant is the key variable characterizing an enzyme.

An example is the effect of statin drugs on the regulatory enzyme of cholesterol synthesis, HMG-CoA reductase

Fig. 3.7.3 Enzyme inhibition: competitive inhibition.

Isoenzymes

Isoenzymes are forms of enzyme that catalyse the same reaction but differ in their structure. For instance, hexokinase and glucokinase are isoenzymes and alkaline phosphatase has distinct bone and liver isoenzymes.

Coenzymes, prosthetic groups and metal ions

Enzymes may contain or interact with small molecules that are not their substrates. Non-covalently bound interacting molecules are coenzymes while prosthetic groups are a structural part of the enzyme:

- coenzymes: NAD^+, $NADP^+$, UTP, CTP, CoA, tetrahydrofolate
- prosthetic groups: FAD, FMN, thiamine pyrophosphate, pyridoxal phosphate, haem.

Inorganic ions participating in enzymatic reactions are called cofactors; manganese, magnesium and calcium ions are common. Vitamins may also act as coenzymes and cofactors (Ch. 8).

Regulation of enzyme activity

Enzyme inhibition. Competitive inhibition (Fig. 3.7.3) is exerted by substances with structures similar to the substrate. It can be reversed by increasing the concentration of substrate. In non-competitive inhibition (Fig. 3.7.4), the inhibitor binds to the enzyme–substrate complex and decreases the maximal velocity (V_{max}) of the reaction (K_m remains unchanged).

Allosterism. Allosteric effectors bind at a site away from the active site and change interactions between enzyme subunits (positive or negative cooperativity), which increases or decreases the affinity of enzyme for that effector itself.

Phosphorylation. The activity of enzymes can be modified by phosphorylation and dephosphorylation, a common mechanism of hormone action (Fig. 3.7.5).

Gene induction and repression. Enzymes may be regulated through controlling transcription of the coding gene. This is usually a longer-term mechanism.

Proteolytic activation. Enzymes may be synthesized as inactive proenzymes and only activated at the site of their action (e.g. the secreted digestive enzymes trypsin and pepsin).

Enzymes as tissue and organ markers

Each tissue possesses a specific set of enzymes. When cells are damaged, enzymes are released. Consequently, measurements of enzyme activities in plasma are widely used as markers of organ damage.

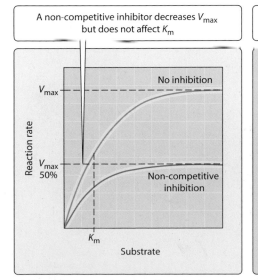

Fig. 3.7.4 Enzyme inhibition: non-competitive inhibition (e.g. the drug omeprazole inhibits the H^+/K^+-ATPase (the proton pump) in the parietal cells of the stomach and the anti-thyroid drugs carbimazole and propylthiouracil inhibit thyroid peroxidase).

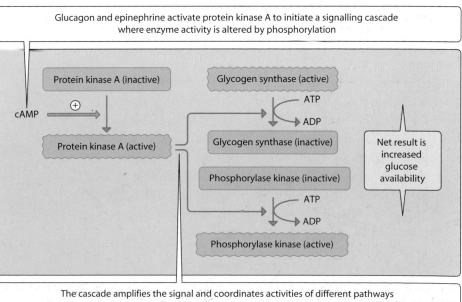
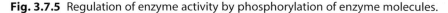

Fig. 3.7.5 Regulation of enzyme activity by phosphorylation of enzyme molecules.

8. Vitamins

Questions
- Why are vitamins important in nutrition?
- What reaction is principally responsible for variation in the concentration of vitamin D in blood in summer and in winter?

Vitamins serve as coenzymes and cofactors for a wide range of enzymes. They are particularly important in energy metabolism, nucleotide synthesis and in antioxidant protection. Deficiencies of folic acid and vitamin B_{12} cause clinically important anaemias.

The most common classification of vitamins is into the fat soluble and the water soluble (Fig. 3.8.1). Unfortunately, the discussion of vitamins in biochemistry textbooks often reads like a telephone directory. The description given below is intended for use as a quick reference rather than for learning details.

Consideration of vitamin status is important in general nutrition and in the formulation of recommendations for healthy eating. Specific assessment of vitamin status may be necessary in malnourished individuals and in those who remain on various forms of nutritional support such as enteral and, particularly, parenteral nutrition.

Fat-soluble vitamins: A, D, E and K

Fat-soluble vitamins are absorbed from the gut in the same manner as fats. Significant quantities are stored so manifestation of deficiencies occurs less quickly than for the water-soluble vitamins and excess intake can be toxic. The water-soluble vitamins are associated with a number of diseases (Table 3.8.1).

Vitamin A

This comprises retinal (retinaldehyde) and retinoic acid structurally related to the carotenoids. Retinyl phosphate participates in the synthesis of mucopolysaccharides and glycoproteins. D-11-*cis*-Retinal is important in vision. Retinoids affect the integrity of epithelial tissue. Vitamin A deficiency is associated with night blindness. However, excess of vitamin A is toxic: it may cause bone pain, dermatitis and hepatosplenomegaly. Dark green and yellow vegetables are a rich source of vitamin A; the animal sources are liver, egg yolk and butter.

Vitamin D

This steroid is essential for calcium and bone metabolism (Fig. 3.8.2). Cholecalciferol is produced in the skin by the irradiation of 7-dehydrocholesterol. Ergocalciferol is vitamin D_2. Both cholecalciferol and ergocalciferol undergo 25-hydroxylation to 25-OH-D_3, which is the main storage form of the vitamin. The 25-OH-D_3 is subject to further hydroxylation in the kidney,

generating the active form of vitamin D, 1,25-$(OH)_2$-D_3. Parathyroid hormone regulates the synthesis of 1,25-$(OH)_2$-D_3. Vitamin D deficiency causes **rickets** in children or **osteomalacia** in adults. Vitamin D, similarly to vitamin A, is toxic in excess, leading to hypercalcaemia and tissue calcification, bone demineralization and also hypercalciuria and kidney stones. The sources of cholecalciferol are fish such as salmon, sardines and herring. It is also present in liver and in egg yolk.

Vitamin E

This comprises several tocopherols, of which α-tocopherol is the most potent. Tocopherols are antioxidants; because of their lipophilicity, they locate in lipid structures, for instance in

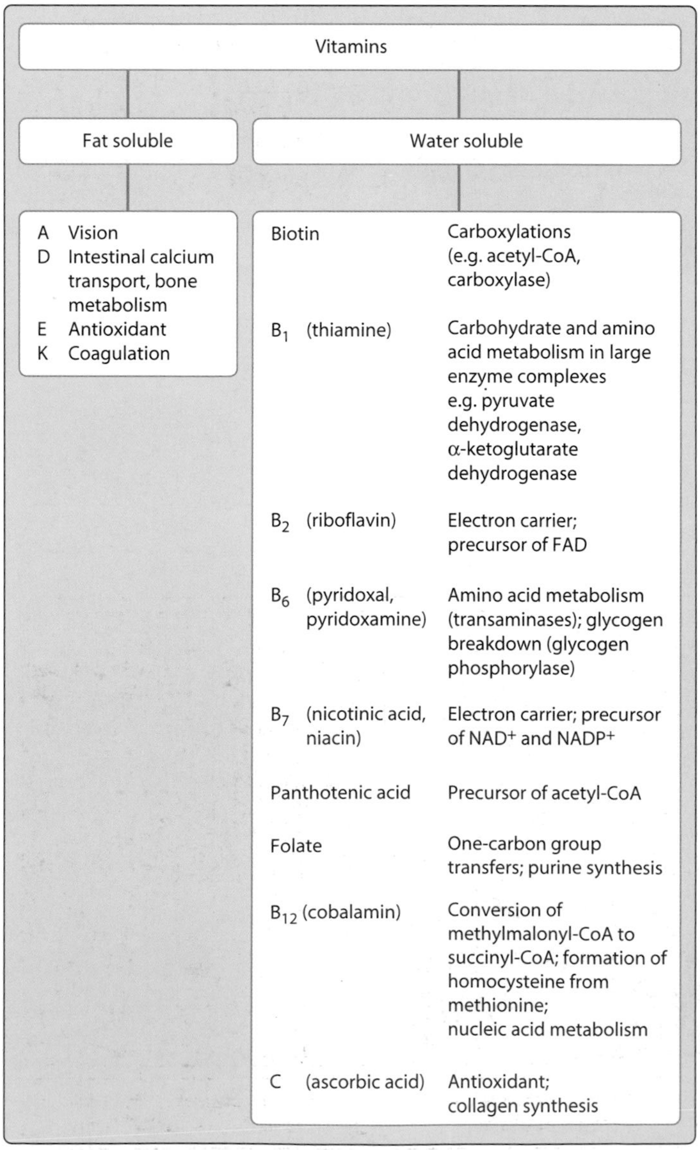

Vitamins		
Fat soluble	**Water soluble**	
A Vision D Intestinal calcium transport, bone metabolism E Antioxidant K Coagulation	Biotin	Carboxylations (e.g. acetyl-CoA, carboxylase)
	B_1 (thiamine)	Carbohydrate and amino acid metabolism in large enzyme complexes e.g. pyruvate dehydrogenase, α-ketoglutarate dehydrogenase
	B_2 (riboflavin)	Electron carrier; precursor of FAD
	B_6 (pyridoxal, pyridoxamine)	Amino acid metabolism (transaminases); glycogen breakdown (glycogen phosphorylase)
	B_7 (nicotinic acid, niacin)	Electron carrier; precursor of NAD^+ and $NADP^+$
	Panthotenic acid	Precursor of acetyl-CoA
	Folate	One-carbon group transfers; purine synthesis
	B_{12} (cobalamin)	Conversion of methylmalonyl-CoA to succinyl-CoA; formation of homocysteine from methionine; nucleic acid metabolism
	C (ascorbic acid)	Antioxidant; collagen synthesis

Fig. 3.8.1 Fat- and water-soluble vitamins.

lipoprotein particles. They protect polyunsaturated fatty acids from oxidation. Epidemiological studies have suggested that vitamin E is protective against cardiovascular disease, but clinical trials to date have failed to confirm this. Vitamin E is widely distributed and vegetable oils are its rich sources.

Vitamin K

This quinone derivative influences the carboxylation of prothrombin and decreases the coagulation time. Vitamin K deficiency can causes defective coagulation and haemorrhage. Vitamin K antagonists such as warfarin are used in clinical practice as anticoagulants. It is present in green leafy vegetables such as cabbage, spinach and broccoli.

Table 3.8.1 THE FAT-SOLUBLE VITAMINS AND DISEASE

Vitamin	Disease	Source
A	Blindness, abortion	Dairy products, fish oils, liver
D	Rickets	Dairy products, fish oils, eggs, sunlight on the skin
E	Infertility	Dairy products, vegetable oils, wheat germ
K	Bleeding in infants	Vegetable oils

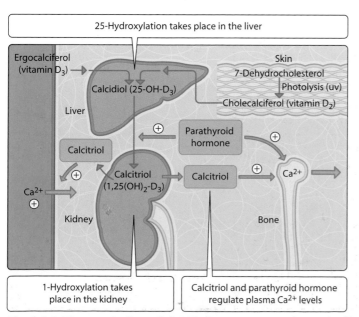

Fig. 3.8.2 The metabolism of vitamin D.

9. Water-soluble vitamins

Questions
■ What are the consequences of vitamin B_1 deficiency?
■ What is the common role of water-soluble vitamins in the body?

Most water-soluble vitamins (with the exception of vitamin B_{12}) cannot be stored long termly in the body. This increases the risk of diet-induced deficiencies. The water-soluble vitamins act as coenzymes. Their lack often causes non-specific symptoms such as dermatitis or diarrhoea and particularly affects tissues undergoing fast growth or regeneration (such as skin), or those with a high energy demand (nerve tissue). Knowledge of the role of vitamins in metabolism has clinical significance when treating patients with inherited defects in critical metabolic pathways. Vitamin therapy is used in those with inborn errors in amino acid catabolism.

Thiamin (vitamin B_1)
The active form of thiamin is thiamin pyrophosphate (TPP). It serves as a coenzyme in carbohydrate, fat and nitrogen metabolism, and in particular is required by complex enzyme systems such as pyruvate dehydrogenase, α-ketoglutarate dehydrogenase and the branched-chain amino acid dehydrogenase. It is also a coenzyme of transketolase, an enzyme participating in the pentose phosphate pathway (the measurement of transketolase in erythrocytes has been used to assess thiamin levels). Thiamin deficiency causes loss of appetite, constipation nausea, mental confusion, ataxia and ophthalmoplegia. The severe form affecting the nervous system is known as the **Wernicke–Korsakoff syndrome**. Severe deficiency causes **beri-beri** (the 'dry' form affecting neuromuscular system and the 'wet' form characterized by oedema). Thiamin is widespread in plant and animal tissues. Grains, legumes, pork and beef are good sources.

Riboflavin
Riboflavin is a component of prosthetic groups involved in electron transfer: FAD and FMN. Its deficiency leads to non-specific symptoms such as **cheilitis** and **glossitis**. The marker used to assess riboflavin is activity of erythrocyte glutathione reductase. It is present in milk, meat, eggs and cereals.

Niacin
Niacin is a component of the electron transfer molecules NAD^+ and $NADP^+$, both synthesized from tryptophan. Their synthesis also requires riboflavin, thiamin and pyridoxine. Deficiency causes **glossitis**, and in severe form manifests itself as **pellagra** with its '3D' symptoms: dermatitis, diarrhoea and dementia. Niacin is present in most foods, particularly in cereal grain, poultry and meat.

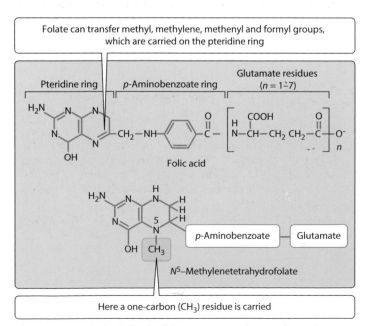

Fig. 3.9.1 Methyltetrahydrofolate serves as donor of 1-carbon residues.

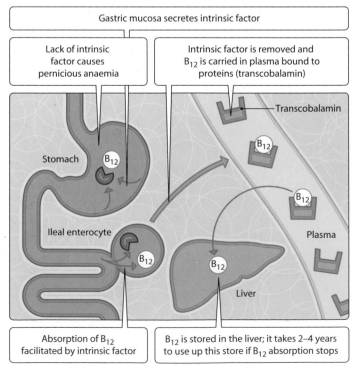

Fig. 3.9.2 The metabolism of vitamin B_{12}.

Pyridoxine (vitamin B_6)

Vitamin B_6 comprises pyridoxine and pyridoxal phosphate. Pyridoxal phosphate serves as coenzyme in transaminases, involved in the metabolism of amino acids. It is also required for glycogen phosphorylase, for the synthesis of D-aminolevulinic acid in the haem synthetic pathway, and for the synthesis of serotonin, norepinephrine and sphingolipids. It is also required for the conversion of homocysteine to cysteine and, as noted above, is a cofactor in the synthesis of NAD^+. Deficiency causes irritability, nervousness and depression and, in severe cases, convulsions. Its sources are meat, vegetables, whole-grain cereals and egg yolks.

Panthotenic acid

Panthotenic acid is a component of coenzyme A and fatty acid synthase. It is widely present in foods and its deficiency has not been demonstrated.

Biotin

This sulphur-containing molecule is the coenzyme of carboxylations. Biotin participates in the reactions of pyruvate carboxylase and propionyl-CoA carboxylase, involved in the metabolism of methionine, leucine and valine. Biotin deficiency may occur in patients treated with parenteral nutrition. Raw egg whites contain the protein avidin, which binds biotin. It is present in peanuts, chocolate and eggs. It is also synthesized by intestinal bacteria.

Folic acid

Folic acid is present in several forms that are polyglutamate derivatives of pteroylmonoglutamic acid (Fig. 3.9.1). Folate is a carrier of methyl groups (it is converted to tetrahydrofolate (THF) by dihydrofolate reductase). It participates in the synthesis of choline, amino acids serine and glycine and, importantly, in the synthesis of purines (dTMP). THF, together with vitamins B_{12} and B_6, is required for the conversion of homocysteine to methionine. Folate deficiency affects purine synthesis. It demonstrates itself as a **macrocytic anaemia**. Folate deficiency may be caused by inadequate intake, defective absorption or an increased demand (the last present during pregnancy and lactation). Folate deficiency in pregnancy leads to **neural tube defects**. It also occurs in **alcoholism** and in **malabsorption syndromes**. Anticonvulsants increase the metabolism of folates. Folate deficiency may also develop in patients treated for cancer with **chemotherapy**. Folic acid is present in most natural foods: the richest sources are yeast, liver and fresh, green, leafy vegetables.

Cobalamin (vitamin B_{12})

This cobalt-containing compound is also known as intrinsic factor; its absorption is dependent upon combination with a protein present in the stomach and known as extrinsic factor (Fig. 3.9.2). Vitamin B_{12} is absorbed in the ileum. It is required for only two reactions: the conversion of homocysteine to methionine, and the conversion of methylmalonyl-CoA to succinyl-CoA in the metabolism of the branched-chain amino acids. Deficiency may occur in strict vegetarians, particularly vegans. The deficiency causes **pernicious anaemia**: a megaloblastic anaemia associated with neurological symptoms (demyelination). Importantly, the availability of cobalamin affects the metabolism of folic acid. This is called the **folate trap**. The reaction:

$$\text{homocysteine} + N^5\text{-methyl-THF} \rightleftharpoons \text{methionine} + \text{THF}$$

regenerates THF from N^5-methyl-THF. If it cannot proceed, folate becomes 'trapped' in the methylated form. Note that the treatment of megaloblastic anaemia with vitamin B_{12} deficiency by folate supplementation alone improves haematological parameters but does not prevent neurological damage. Vitamin B_{12} is present in meats, particularly liver.

Vitamin C (ascorbic acid)

Vitamin C is a reducing agent and an antioxidant. It participates in hydroxylation reactions and is particularly important for the hydroxylation of lysine and proline in protocollagen. It affects wound healing and bone formation, and deficiency may cause haemorrhages and anaemia. Severe deficiency leads to **scurvy**. It is present in fruit and vegetables, particularly in citrus fruits.

EFFECTS OF A DIETARY DEFICIENCY

A 28-year-old woman who had been taking a vegan diet for 5 years complained of excessive tiredness and appeared pale. Her haemoglobin concentration was low and the erythrocytes were increased in size (macrocytosis). There were no neurological symptoms but her blood vitamin B_{12} concentration was low.

Since the sources of B_{12} are animal products, the strict vegan diet can lead to vitamin B_{12} deficiency.

10. Endocrine regulation of metabolism: general features

Questions
- What is understood by the hierarchical organization of the endocrine system?
- How is osmolality controlled?

Hormones are macroregulators of metabolism (Fig. 3.10.1). This is particularly well illustrated by the example of insulin and glucagon, which in a comprehensive manner regulate carbohydrate, fat and nitrogen metabolism. Disorders of the endocrine system can give rise to effects at multiple metabolic pathways and affected multiple organ systems. More detailed discussion of endocrine syndromes is beyond the scope of this book. Table 3.10.1 shows the most important syndromes.

Chemically, there are two main types of hormone: proteins and steroids. Some hormones, such as thyroxine, and some neurotransmitters, such as epinephrine or norepinephrine, are amino acid derivatives. A broader definition of hormones would also include factors that exert paracrine and autocrine action, such as cytokines and growth factors.

Hierarchical organization of the endocrine system

The endocrine system is organized in a hierarchical manner (Fig. 3.10.2).

Hypothalamus

Importantly, the highest level of control, the hypothalamus, integrates the physical and emotional signals, providing a major gateway for the central nervous system (CNS) influence on metabolic responses. The hypothalamus controls pituitary–adrenal, pituitary–thyroid and pituitary–gonadal axes through the production of releasing factors. It also directly controls water excretion through the secretion of vasopressin (antidiuretic hormone (ADH)), which is synthesized in the hypothalamic nuclei and transported along the axons to the posterior pituitary. Vasopressin secretion is controlled primarily by plasma osmolality (through hypothalamic osmoreceptors) and by plasma volume (see p. 000).

The hypothalamic releasing factors that control the anterior pituitary are corticotrophin-releasing hormone (CRH), thyrotrophin-releasing hormone (TRH), growth hormone-releasing hormone (GHRH) and gonadotrophin-releasing hormone (GnRH). Growth hormone secretion is inhibited by somatostatin.

The pituitary

The **anterior pituitary**, in turn, controls secretion of endocrine glands that produce 'effector' hormones. Adrenocorticotrophic hormone (ACTH, corticotrophin) stimulates secretion of the adrenal steroid hormones except aldosterone (aldosterone is controlled by the renin–angiotensin system). ACTH is derived from a larger peptide, proopiomelanocortin (POMC). The hydrolysis produces β-lipotrophin which is a precursor of endorphins. The secretion of anterior pituitary hormones exhibits diurnal rhythm (ACTH).

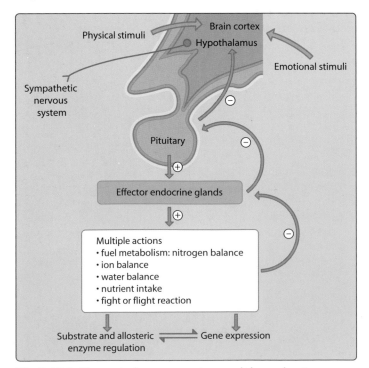

Fig. 3.10.1 The central nervous system and the endocrine system.

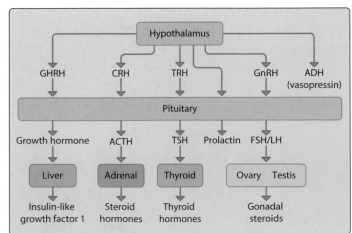

Fig. 3.10.2 Hierarchical organization of the endocrine system. (See text for abbreviations.)

Thyroid-stimulating hormone (TSH), acting through adenylyl cyclase, controls the thyroid gland. The glycoprotein hormones follicle-stimulating hormone (FSH) and luteinizing hormone (LH) regulate the function of ovaries and testes. The 'odd-man-out' is prolactin, which, rather than controlling an endocrine gland, directly regulates secretion of breast milk. Growth hormone (GH), secreted by the acidophilic cells in the anterior pituitary, is a major anabolic hormone acting through insulin growth factors (IGF-1 and IGF-2).

The gonadotrophins FSH and LH regulate the development of ovarian follicles (FSH) and ovulation and ovarian synthesis of oestrogens and progesterone (LH). Their secretion is determined by complex feedback mechanisms during the menstrual cycle. In men, FSH controls the development of seminiferous tubules in the testis, and LH stimulates testosterone secretion.

The hypothalamic–pituitary–effector axes contain multiple levels of control, both by feedback inhibition and neural stimuli. Usually, the effector hormone suppresses both pituitary and hypothalamic secretion. Pituitary hormones also inhibit the hypothalamic releasing factors.

Parathyroid

The parathyroid gland secretes parathyroid hormone (parathormone, PTH). PTH acts in concert with calcitonin, secreted by the thyroid, and the steroid vitamin D to control calcium and phosphate homeostasis and bone metabolism. A major regulator of PTH is plasma calcium ion concentration (see also Ch. 8).

The pancreas: insulin and glucagon

Insulin and glucagon regulate fuel utilization, affecting predominantly carbohydrate and lipid metabolism. Insulin also stimulates protein synthesis. Insulin and glucagon are not under pituitary control. The main regulators of their secretion are ingested fuels: primarily glucose, but also amino acids and fatty acids.

The adrenal glands

The adrenal cortex secretes steroid hormones. These have two main roles: a permissive role, facilitating the action of other hormones in the resting state; and an active response to a threatening change whether external or internal, such as disease (see Ch. 11). The adrenal medulla produces the biogenic amines (Ch. 13).

The gonads

The gonads produce steroid hormones (Ch. 12).

The thyroid

The thyroid gland produces the amino acid-derived thyroid hormones (Ch. 13).

Table 3.10.1 THE MOST IMPORTANT ENDOCRINE DISORDERS

Clinical entity	Hormone involved	Type of disorder
Dwarfism	Growth hormone	Deficiency
Gigantism/acromegaly	Growth hormone (before/after adolescence)	Excess
Diabetes insipidus	Vasopressin (ADH)	Deficiency
Syndrome of inappropriate ADH secretion (SIADH)	Vasopressin (ADH)	Excess
Hypothyroidism	Thyroid hormones	Deficiency
Hyperthyroidism	Thyroid hormones	Excess
Hypoparathyroidism	Parathyroid hormone	Deficiency
Hyperparathyroidism	Parathyroid hormone	Excess
Cushing syndrome	Primarily adrenal glucocorticoids Cushing's disease: ACTH	Excess
Addison's disease	Glucocorticoids	Deficiency
Diabetes mellitus	Insulin	Deficiency or resistance to
Hypogonadism and infertility	Pituitary, ovarian or testicular hormones	Various disorders
Phaeochromocytoma	Catecholamines	Excess

11. Mechanisms of hormone action and endocrine dysregulation

Questions
- The action of which pituitary hormone involves adenylyl cyclase?
- What is the role of the receptor in the action of steroid hormones?
- Why are the so-called dynamic function tests important in the diagnosis of endocrine diseases?

Peptide hormones cannot cross cell membranes (Fig. 3.11.1). Their signals are mediated by membrane receptors, protein structures embedded into membranes that bind hormones in a specific fashion.

The binding of hormones to receptors triggers intracellular signalling cascades. The signalling pathways involve phosphorylation of receptors themselves, interaction of low-molecular-weight proteins (**G-proteins**) with GTP and GDP and the generation of a 'classic' second messenger, **cAMP**, by adenylyl cyclase (Ch. 7). Formation of cAMP, in turn, stimulates **protein kinase A**, which initiates an enzymatic cascade of phosphorylations involving an array of other protein kinases and phosphatases. The products of these phosphorylations then phosphorylate other 'effector' enzymes. An important class of signalling molecules, **diacylglycerols** and **phosphatidylinositols**, are produced from membrane phospholipids by phospholipase. These are hydrophobic and disseminate their signal travelling within the membrane lipid bilayer. This pathway is linked with changes in the concentration of intracellular calcium ions.

Mechanism of action of steroid hormones
Steroids act in a different manner to protein hormones. Like cholesterol, steroids are lipid soluble and can cross biological membranes (Fig. 3.11.2). In the cytoplasm, they bind to their protein receptors. Steroid hormone receptors are ligand-activated transcription factors that possess DNA-binding domains (e.g. the zinc finger motif). The binding of a steroid activates the receptor, and the steroid–receptor complex transfers into the nucleus. In the nucleus, the complex binds to an appropriate DNA-response element and modifies transcription.

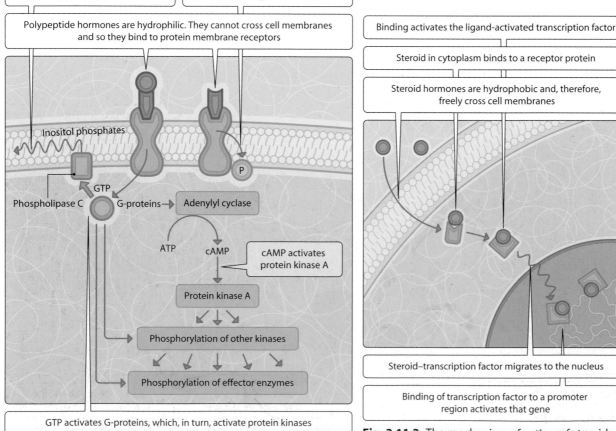

Phosphoinositol phosphate signalling pathway in membrane

Receptor phosphorylates itself on binding of hormone

Polypeptide hormones are hydrophilic. They cannot cross cell membranes and so they bind to protein membrane receptors

Inositol phosphates

GTP

Phospholipase C — G-proteins → Adenylyl cyclase

ATP   cAMP   cAMP activates protein kinase A

Protein kinase A

Phosphorylation of other kinases

Phosphorylation of effector enzymes

GTP activates G-proteins, which, in turn, activate protein kinases

Fig. 3.11.1 The mechanism of action of polypeptide hormones.

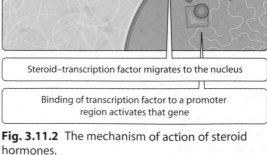

Binding activates the ligand-activated transcription factor

Steroid in cytoplasm binds to a receptor protein

Steroid hormones are hydrophobic and, therefore, freely cross cell membranes

Steroid–transcription factor migrates to the nucleus

Binding of transcription factor to a promoter region activates that gene

Fig. 3.11.2 The mechanism of action of steroid hormones.

Causes of endocrine dysregulation

Endocrine disorders may be caused by hormone excess, hormone deficiency or by tissue resistance to a hormone. Tissue resistance may be caused by

- plasma antibodies to a hormone: pre-receptor resistance
- abnormalities of a hormone receptor: receptor resistance
- defects in the signalling system: post-receptor resistance.

Post-receptor mechanisms affecting the intracellular signalling systems are most important. Importantly, hypo- or hypersecretion may occur at any of the regulatory levels: the effector gland, the pituitary or the hypothalamus.

Investigation of the endocrine system

Endocrine investigations involve measurements of hormone concentration in plasma. This could mean single measurements or multiple sampling to assess, for instance, the presence or absence of a diurnal rhythm (cortisol in the diagnosis of adrenal hyperfunction). Known regulatory feedback mechanisms are extensively exploited in function tests, which help to diagnose disorders associated with deficiency or excess of a hormone (Fig. 3.11.3).

Syndromes of excess and deficiency of adrenal steroids

Deficiency of adrenal steroids (adrenal failure). This is known as **Addison's disease** and is most commonly of autoimmune origin but may be secondary to pituitary disease. It is characterized by lethargy and weakness, leading to weight loss, hyperpigmentation and postural hypotension. Hypovolaemic shock may develop in the acute adrenal crisis.

Adrenal crisis as a medical emergency. The diagnosis of severe adrenal failure is based on a function test known as the **Synacthen test**; this measures cortisol concentration before and after an injection of synthetic ACTH (Fig. 3.11.4).

Excess of adrenal steroids. Excess of adrenal steroids is known as **Cushing syndrome**, or **Cushing's disease** if the cause lies in the pituitary. It results in a central distribution of body fat, a typical 'moon' face and concomitant muscle wasting. Hypertension is common and so is glucose intolerance. Biochemically, this is characterized by increased concentration of cortisol, and the loss of normal diurnal rhythm (higher concentration in the morning and lower at night). Patients with Cushing syndrome will show lack of cortisol suppression after administration of another steroid, dexamethasone.

FUNCTION TEST TO DIAGNOSE ADRENAL INSUFFICIENCY

A 48-year-woman was admitted to the hospital confused after a short term 'flu-like illness. She appeared to be severely ill: she was in shock and had oliguria and a pigmented face. Laboratory results showed severe hyperkalaemia and hyponatraemia. A Synacthen test (Fig. 3.11.4) showed low cortisol concentration and lack of increase in cortisol after Synacthen. Adrenal insufficiency (Addison's disease) was diagnosed. She was given hydrocortisone and intravenous fluids. The Addisonian crisis is a medical emergency and may be precipitated, as it was in this case, by infection, and also by trauma or surgery.

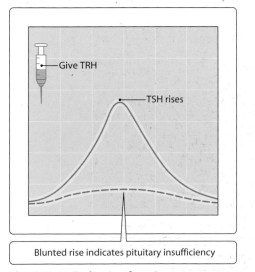

Blunted rise indicates pituitary insufficiency

Fig. 3.11.3 Endocrine function tests. TRH, thyrotrophin-releasing hormone; TSH, thyroid-stimulating hormone.

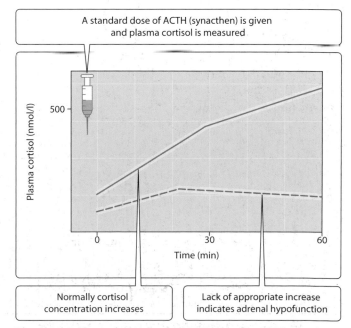

A standard dose of ACTH (synacthen) is given and plasma cortisol is measured

Normally cortisol concentration increases

Lack of appropriate increase indicates adrenal hypofunction

Fig. 3.11.4 Cortisol response to ACTH is a diagnostic test in adrenal hypofunction.

12. Regulation of metabolism by steroid hormones

Questions
■ What is the anatomical target of aldosterone in the kidney?
■ What is the medical emergency associated with impaired adrenal function?

Steroid hormones are structurally derived from cholesterol and include adrenal and gonadal steroids and vitamin D. They contribute to the control of energy metabolism, particularly during stress (glucocorticoids have an anti-insulin effect); electrolyte metabolism; and affect growth, sexual maturation and fertility. The secretion of most of the steroid hormones is controlled by the endocrine axes involving hypothalamic and pituitary polypeptide hormones (Fig. 3.12.1).

Metabolism of steroid hormones

Synthesis and transport

The original precursor of all steroids is acetyl-CoA, and, downstream in the synthetic pathway, **pregnenolone** is the common precursor of the adrenal steroids (Fig. 3.12.2). There are four main classes of adrenal steroid: mineralocorticoids (i.e. aldosterone), glucocorticoids (cortisol), oestrogens (oestriol) and androgens (testosterone). Steroids are often transported in blood bound to proteins such as cortisol-binding globulin (CBG) or sex-hormone-binding globulin (SHBG).

Removal

Humans cannot metabolize the steroid ring. Therefore, steroid hormones are usually conjugated with glucuronide before being excreted in urine.

Adrenal steroids

Glucocorticoids (cortisol and corticosterone). Glucocorticoids (cortisol being the principal one in humans) are the group of steroids with the most direct metabolic action. Cortisol is one of the principal anti-insulin hormones. It exerts a hyperglycaemic action, stimulating gluconeogenesis, lipolysis and proteolysis. Along with epinephrine, cortisol is one of the main hormones secreted during chronic stress. Cortisol secretion remains under the control of ACTH.

Mineralocorticoids (aldosterone). Mineralocorticoids secreted by the adrenal cortex regulate electrolyte balance. Aldosterone, the principal mineralocorticoid, controls the reabsorption of sodium and potassium ions in the distal tubules of the kidney. Together with vasopressin, which regulates renal water excretion, they constitute the comprehensive system controlling the volume and composition of the extracellular fluid (Ch. 6).

Oestrogens and progesterone. The oestrogens and progesterone remain under pituitary gonadotrophin control and regulate the menstrual cycle. Oestrogens also contribute to growth and differentiation, being responsible for the development of secondary female characteristics.

Androgens. The androgens are anabolic. Dehydroepiandrosterone (DHEA) and dehydroepiandrosterone sulphate (DHEAS) are the main adrenal androgens. Testosterone is synthesized in testes and ovaries but not in the adrenal cortex.

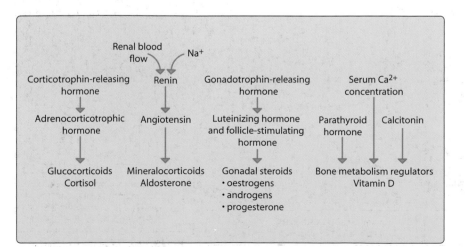

Fig. 3.12.1 Systems involved in the control of steroid hormone secretion.

Vitamin D

Vitamin D, under the control of parathyroid hormone (PTH) and calcitonin, controls calcium and phosphate homeostasis and bone metabolism. PTH regulates synthesis of $1,25\text{-}(OH)_2\text{-}D_3$ (see Ch. 8).

Disorders of steroid synthesis

The interdependent pathways of steroid synthesis allow rare defects in steroid synthesis to be identified by profiling. The most common inherited disorder of steroid hormone metabolism is **21-hydroxylase deficiency**. The diagnosis of deficiency is made by identifying an excess of steroid metabolite, which accumulates upstream of the point of enzymatic defect: in this case 17α-hydroxyprogesterone (Fig. 3.12.3).

TREATMENT OF HIGH BLOOD PRESSURE

A 57-year-old woman presented with blood pressure of 170/95 and 168/97 mmHg (recommended values below 140/80 mmHg) while being treated with a diuretic for hypertension. Retinal changes were noted on optical fundus examination. She was prescribed an additional hypotensive agent, an angiotensin-converting enzyme (ACE) inhibitor. After 2 weeks, her blood pressure had decreased to 145/88 mmHg.

The ACE inhibitors block conversion of angiotensinogen to angiotensin II (the most potent vasoconstrictor known) in the renin–angiotensin–aldosterone system. The angiotensin receptor antagonists (e.g. losartan) block angiotensin action at target cells. Both types of drug are effective in the treatment of hypertension and cardiac failure. Retinal changes, deterioration of renal function and cardiac left ventricular hypertrophy are all signs of hypertensive organ damage.

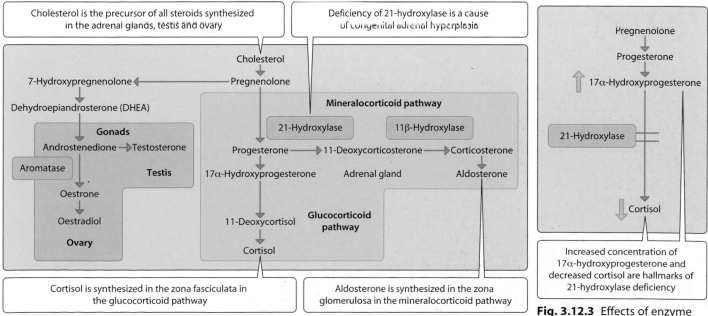

Fig. 3.12.2 The synthesis of steroid hormones.

Fig. 3.12.3 Effects of enzyme deficiency in a pathway.

13. Amino acid-derived hormones and neurotransmitters

Questions
- How are biogenic amines defined?
- Which is the biologically active form of the thyroid hormone?
- What is the difference between ionotropic and metabotropic receptors for neurotransmitters?

Amino acids are precursors of thyroid hormones and of some neurotransmitters. One of the neurotransmitters, epinephrine, plays a major role in fuel metabolism, controlling the fight-and-flight response, in addition to its role in nerve transmission.

Thyroid hormones
Thyroxine is an anabolic hormone secreted by the thyroid gland. It is an effector hormone in the hypothalamic–pituitary–thyroid axis. The hypothalamus secretes thyrotrophin-releasing hormone (TRH), which acts on the pituitary to stimulate secretion of thyroid-stimulating hormone (TSH); this, in turn, stimulates the thyroid.

Thyroid hormones are synthesized from tyrosine, which is generated from the essential amino acid phenylalanine (note

that defective conversion of phenylalanine into tyrosine causes **phenylketonuria**; Fig. 3.13.1). Thyroid hormone synthesis requires dietary iodine (dietary deficiencies of iodine, now rare, may cause hypothyroidism). Iodine is converted to iodide in the stomach and is actively taken up from the bloodstream by the thyroid gland. It is then oxidized by thyroperoxidase. The same enzyme incorporates iodide into tyrosine residues while they are part of the side chains of a thyroid protein, thyroglobulin. This produces monoiodotyrosine (MIT) and diiodotyrosine (DIT). Subsequently, MIT and DIT pair in different combinations yielding either thyroxine (two DIT molecules give tetraiodothyronine (T_4)) or triodothyronine (one MIT and one DIT give T_3). Subsequently, lysosomal proteases release the hormones from thyroglobulin. In target tissues, T_4 is converted to T_3. Remaining MIT and DIT are deiodinated by deiodinase.

The action of thyroxine
Thyroid hormones are anabolic and affect fuel metabolism as well as growth and cell differentiation. They increase basal metabolic rate and thus play an important role in thermogenesis. Thyroid hormones act through the cytoplasmic (non-membrane) receptors similar to the steroid receptors, and affect gene expression through DNA-response elements.

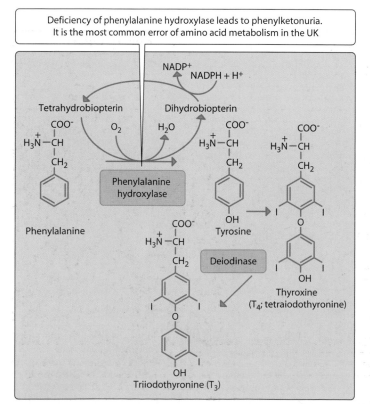

Fig. 3.13.1 Phenylalanine, tyrosine and thyroid hormones.

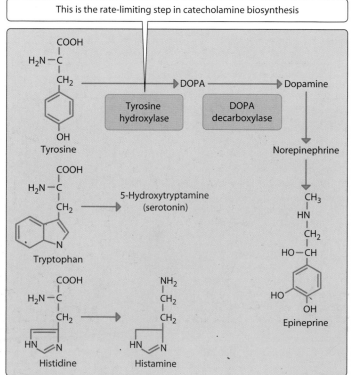

Fig. 3.13.2 The biogenic amines.

Biogenic amines

Biogenic amines are derivatives of aromatic amino acids (Fig. 3.13.2). The catecholamines are **epinephrine**, **norepinephrine** and **dopamine**. They are synthesized from tyrosine. Other biogenic amines are **serotonin** (5-hydroxytryptamine) derived from tryptophan, and **histamine** derived from histidine. Other compounds in this group that act as neurotransmitters include **glutamate**, **aspartate**, **glycine** (–), and **γ-aminobutyric acid** (GABA).

Nature of neurotransmitters

Neurotransmitters are chemical messengers of the nerve cells (Fig. 3.13.3). Epinephrine is secreted by the adrenal medulla as a hormone that affects both parasympathetic and sympathetic functions. In the peripheral nervous system, the most important neurotransmitters are norepinephrine and lipid-derived **acetylcholine**. Both are synthesized in neurons. Norepinephrine serves as a neurotransmitter in the sympathetic nerves and acetylcholine (Fig. 3.13.3) in skeletal muscle. Acetylcholine ($CH_3–CO–O–CH_2–CH_2–N^+–(CH_3)_3$) is synthesized from acetyl-CoA and choline by choline acetyltransferase. Acetylcholine is degraded by acetylcholinesterase to acetate and choline. Acetylcholine is a neurotransmitter in preganglionic nerves and in the postganglionic parasympathetic ones. Other neurotransmitters derived from amino acids such as GABA (inhibitory neurotransmitter), and glutamate, act in the CNS. Peptide neurotransmitters include the **opioid peptides** (endorphins, enkephalins and dynorphin) and cholecystokinin.

Neurotransmitter receptors

Neurotransmitters act on either ionotropic or metabotropic receptors (Fig. 3.13.3). Ionotropic receptors are ion channels, and metabotropic receptors, such as the adrenoceptor, are membrane-spanning proteins linked to the signalling system protein hormones. Therefore, catecholamines act through the G-protein, adenylyl cyclase, protein kinases system and through calcium channels.

Degradation of neurotransmitters

After secretion at the synapse, catecholamines are metabolized by monoamine oxidase (MAO) and catechol-O-methyltransferase. Norepinephrine and epinephrine are metabolized to vanillylmandelic acid (VMA) and dopamine is metabolized to homovanillic acid. Acetylcholine is degraded by acetylcholinesterase. Some of the 'used' neurotransmitter may be taken back up by the nerve cell (this is known as reuptake).

CATECHOLAMINE-SECRETING TUMOURS

A 55-year-old woman complained of occasional headaches, palpitations and sweating, which 24-hour ambulatory monitoring of blood pressure showed were associated with bouts of hypertension reaching 220/120 mmHg. There were high concentrations of catecholamine metabolites in urine and subsequent renal imaging showed an adrenal mass. This was surgically removed and histology revealed it to be a catecholamine-secreting benign phaeochromocytoma.

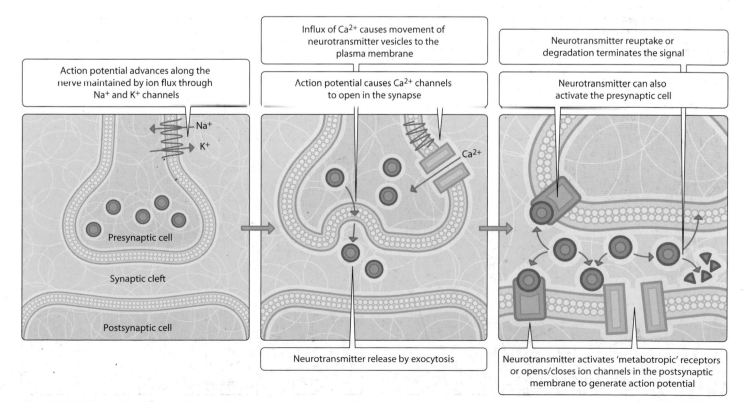

Fig. 3.13.3 The action of neurotransmitters.

14. Cellular signalling

Questions
- What is the role of G-proteins in hormone action?
- Which signalling cascade involves changes in the intra-cellular calcium concentration?
- How are membrane phospholipids associated with endocrine signalling?

Signalling pathways transmit information from hormone or neurotransmitter molecules to target molecules. They operate on a cascade principle, which enables systemic effects to be exerted rapidly and from minute amounts of hormones. Each subsequent step produces a multiplied response, mostly through the involvement of enzymes (Fig. 3.14.1).

Types of signalling event

Binding of a ligand to its receptor
Peptide hormones and epinephrine bind to membrane-spanning proteins, the receptors, inducing changes in the receptor and, in some cases causing its autophosphorylation. Activated receptor activates small proteins called G-proteins and initiates the cascades.

The cAMP pathway
The cAMP signalling cascade (Fig. 3.14.2) is triggered by G-proteins, which are activated on binding GTP (Fig. 3.14.3) and may be stimulatory or inhibitory. The stimulatory ones activate adenylyl cyclase, which produces cAMP; this activates the

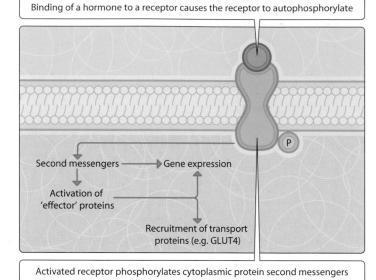

Fig. 3.14.1 Signalling system based on hormone receptor autophosphorylation and phosphorylation of downstream proteins.

cAMP-dependent protein kinase (also known as protein kinase A (PKA)) to initiate further protein phosphorylation cascades.

The inositol phosphate pathway
The G-proteins also activate phospholipase C (PLC), which degrades membrane phospholipids producing inositol phosphates, including inositol 1,4,5-trisphosphate (IP$_3$), and diacyl-

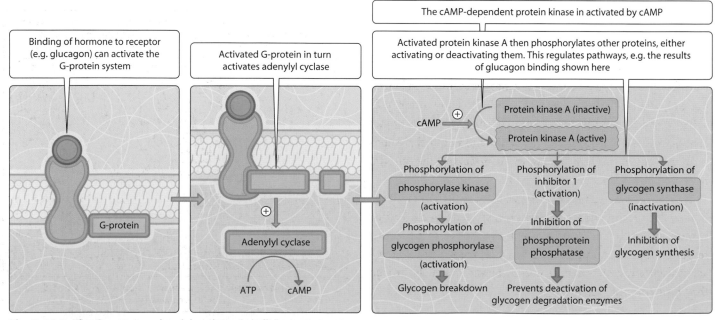

Fig. 3.14.2 The G-protein–adenylyl cyclase signalling system.

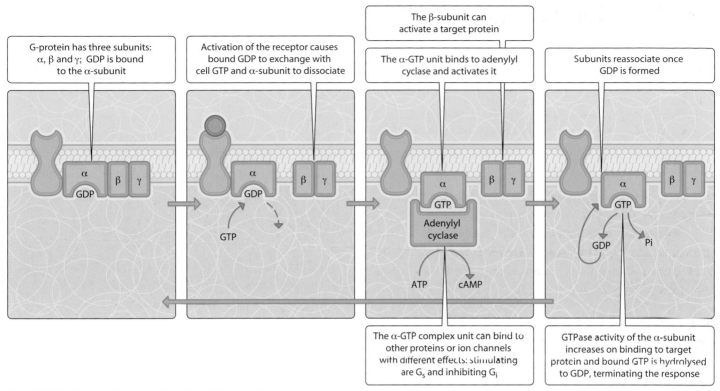

G-protein has three subunits: α, β and γ; GDP is bound to the α-subunit

Activation of the receptor causes bound GDP to exchange with cell GTP and α-subunit to dissociate

The β-subunit can activate a target protein

The α-GTP unit binds to adenylyl cyclase and activates it

Subunits reassociate once GDP is formed

The α-GTP complex unit can bind to other proteins or ion channels with different effects: stimulating are G$_s$ and inhibiting G$_i$

GTPase activity of the α-subunit increases on binding to target protein and bound GTP is hydrolysed to GDP, terminating the response

Fig. 3.14.3 The mechanism of action of G-proteins.

glycerol (DAG) (Fig. 3.14.4). This triggers an increase in intracellular Ca^{2+} concentration, which, with DAG, activates protein kinase C, leading to phosphorylation of other enzyme molecules.

Protein phosphorylation

The phosphorylation of proteins by metabolic kinases and their dephosphorylation by phosphatases is a major metabolic regulatory mechanism (see Chs 31 and 32).

Receptor types

The adrenoceptors

Adrenoceptors bind epinephrine and norepinephrine and affect not only fuel metabolism but also cardiac, vascular and pulmonary function, including blood pressure. Catecholamines complement the action of insulin and glucagon on fuel metabolism and are particularly important in inducing the survival response to trauma and stress.

There are several classes of adrenoceptor. Adenylyl cyclase is inhibited by stimulation of α$_2$-adrenoceptors and activated by stimulation of β$_1$- and β$_2$-adrenoceptors. The β$_1$-adrenoceptors respond both to norepinephrine and epinephrine. The α$_2$-adrenoceptor responds to norepinephrine and to signals through the phosphoinositol pathway.

Steroid hormone receptors

As steroid hormones can enter the cell freely, they bind to cytoplasmic receptors. These complexes move to the nucleus to alter gene activity; consequently the response is slower than with peptide hormones (Ch. 11).

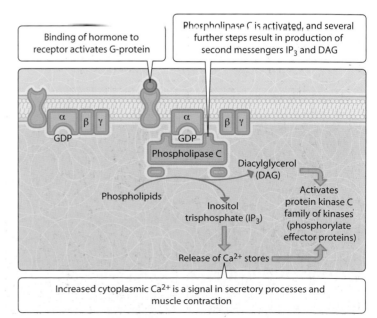

Binding of hormone to receptor activates G-protein

Phospholipase C is activated, and several further steps result in production of second messengers IP$_3$ and DAG

Phospholipids

Diacylglycerol (DAG)

Activates protein kinase C family of kinases (phosphorylate effector proteins)

Inositol trisphosphate (IP$_3$)

Release of Ca^{2+} stores

Increased cytoplasmic Ca^{2+} is a signal in secretory processes and muscle contraction

Fig. 3.14.4 The phosphatidylinositol signalling pathway.

15. Haemoglobin and oxygen delivery to tissues

Questions
- How do the dissociation curves of haemoglobin A and haemoglobin F differ?
- What level of 2,3-bisphosphoglycerate would you expect during a climb in the Himalayas?
- Which laboratory test best defines respiratory failure?

Oxygen supply is a prerequisite for biological oxidations. It is delivered to cells by a metalloprotein, haemoglobin. Oxygen delivery is closely linked to the hydrogen ion (acid–base) balance.

Iron metabolism
The human body contains 4–5 g iron in either the ferrous (Fe^{2+}) or ferric (Fe^{3+}) form. The so-called non-haem iron is present in, for instance, iron–sulphur complexes in the respiratory chain. Iron is an important catalyst of redox reactions (e.g. the reduction of ribonucleotides to deoxyribonucleotides). It also activates O_2 to produce the superoxide anion. In the blood, iron is bound to transferrin. It is stored in association with proteins, ferritin and haemosiderin.

Haemoglobin and oxygen delivery
Delivery of O_2 to tissues relies on an efficient protein carrier: the haemoglobin present in erythrocytes. There is around 950 g haemoglobin in a human body. Haemoglobin is a tetrameric protein possessing two α- and β-chains. Its molecular mass is 65 500 Da, and it has four haem groups. In the haem ring, the ferrous (Fe^{2+}) iron is bound to two histidine residues (Fig. 3.15.1).

Modulation of oxygen binding
The α- and β-chains in deoxyhaemoglobin remain in the so-called tight conformation (the T-form) whereas oxyhaemoglobin represents a relaxed R-form, with a higher affinity to O_2. The quarternary structure of haemoglobin and thus its ability to bind O_2 can be modified by allosteric effectors, the most important of which are 2,3-bisphosphoglycerate (2,3-BPG) and hydrogen ions (Fig. 3.15.2).

The role of 2,3-bisphosphoglycerate
2,3-Bisphosphoglycerate (a by-product of glycolysis) is synthesized from 1,3-bisphosphoglycerate. It is a negative allosteric effector that decreases the affinity of haemoglobin for O_2 and promotes the dissociation of oxyhaemoglobin (Fig. 3.15.3). Its binding to the deoxyhaemoglobin β-chain stabilizes the deoxy-

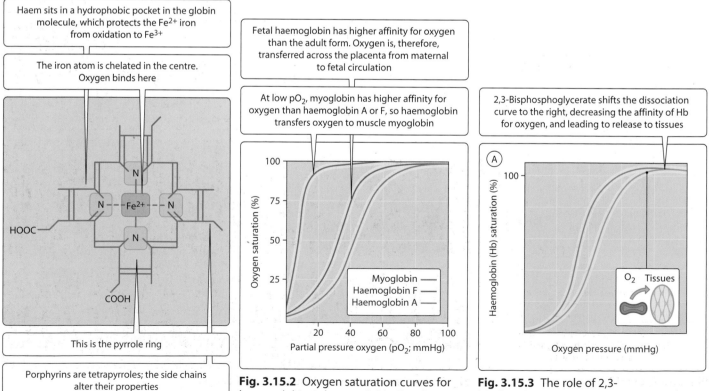

Fig. 3.15.1 The structure of haem.

Fig. 3.15.2 Oxygen saturation curves for haemoglobin A, haemoglobin F and myoglobin.

Fig. 3.15.3 The role of 2,3-bisphosphoglycerate and pH.

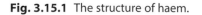

genated state. This maintains the ability of haemoglobin to dissociate maximal amount of O_2 in tissues, even at lower partial pressures of O_2. The concentration of 2,3-BPG increases with a decrease in O_2 tension such as during work at high altitude.

The effect of pH: the Bohr effect

The Bohr effect is the alteration of the haemoglobin dissociation curve by pH (Fig. 3.15.3). It is linked to CO_2 transport. When carbonic acid forms in tissues, it dissociates into hydrogen and bicarbonate ions. The hydrogen ion binds to haemoglobin and this decreases haemoglobin affinity for O_2, and so O_2 is released to the tissues. In the lungs, hydrogen ions are released from haemoglobin, which will facilitate the release of CO_2 from bicarbonate and lead to an increase in the affinity of haemoglobin for O_2.

Fetal haemoglobin

Fetal haemoglobin (HbF; Fig. 3.13.2) has higher affinity for O_2 than adult haemoglobin. This assists movement of O_2 across the placenta.

Mutatant haemoglobin chains

Over 150 mutations that affect haemoglobin chains exist, many changing the affinity of haemoglobin for O_2. The most important clinically are the ones that lead to **sickle cell anaemia** (the presence of haemoglobin S), and to **thalassaemia** (in β-thalassaemia, no β-chains are synthesized).

Conditions characterized by hypoxia

The most important laboratory marker of O_2 delivery is the partial pressure of O_2 in the arterial blood (pO_2). Figure 3.15.4 illustrates the major causes of hypoxia and tissue ischaemia.

RESPIRATORY FAILURE

The pO_2 is the most important indicator of respiratory failure. During a severe asthmatic attack, pO_2 is low and pCO_2 is also usually low because of hyperventilation. It may, however, increase in a severe prolonged asthmatic attack.

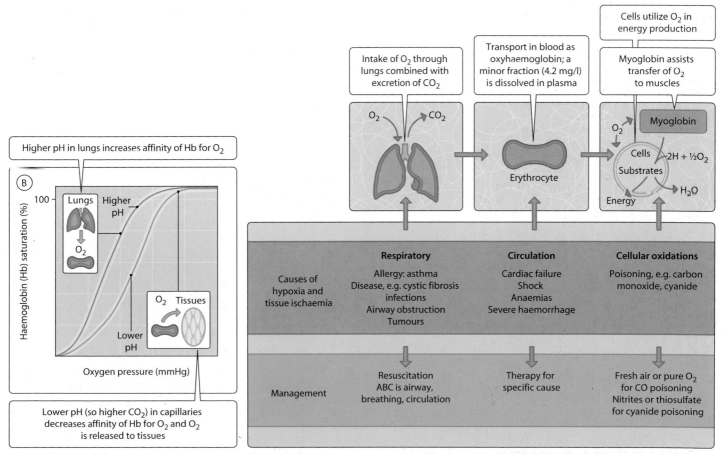

Fig. 3.15.3, cont'd

Fig. 3.15.4 The transport and metabolism of oxygen.

16. Amino acids I

Questions
- What is a zwitterion?
- How are amino acids joined together in chains?

Amino acids are the building blocks of proteins. They contain nitrogen in the form of amino groups. They also serve as substrates for the synthesis of other nitrogen-containing compounds such as nucleosides and haem, and are precursors of a number of specialized hormone and neurotransmitter molecules. They serve as metabolic fuel in catabolic states such as starvation or trauma.

Importantly, the body does not store amino acids. The excess nitrogen is converted to urea in the liver and excreted. However, there is a 'reserve' of amino acids, the muscle protein, which is used for energy in case of need. Naturally, there are limits to the utilization of this resource: excessive muscle wasting, particularly if it affects respiratory muscles, is harmful. Therefore, there are metabolic mechanisms that spare muscle protein in catabolic conditions.

The structure of amino acids

The diverse structure of amino acids is the basis for the diversity of proteins. Amino acids possess in their structure at least one carboxyl and one amino group (Fig. 3.16.1). All except glycine have an asymmetric carbon: a carbon that is bonded to four different chemical residues. Consequently, they form so-called hybrid ions (**zwitterions**). This means that at the physiological pH they may at the same time possess positively charged (amino) and negatively charged (carboxyl) residues: they are amphoteric (Fig. 3.16.1).

Amino acids are characterized by **stereoisomerism**. This means that their residues can be spatially arranged around the asymmetric carbon atom in different ways. Stereoisomerism affects the optical characteristics of a molecule. The amino acids, much the same as sugars, exist in D and L forms. The amino acids found in proteins are L-stereoisomers.

Twenty amino acids are coded in the genetic code. However, many more can be formed by post-translational modifications. For example, 4-hydroxyproline and 5-hydroxylysine are commonly found in collagen, and ornithine and citrulline participate in the urea cycle.

The diversity of amino acids results from differences in the properties of their side chains (Table 3.16.1 and Ch. 17).

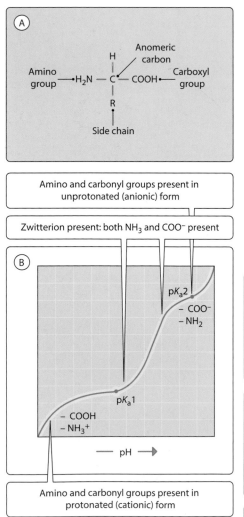

Amino and carbonyl groups present in unprotonated (anionic) form

Zwitterion present: both NH_3 and COO^- present

Amino and carbonyl groups present in protonated (cationic) form

Fig. 3.16.1 The basic structure and ionization of an amino acid.

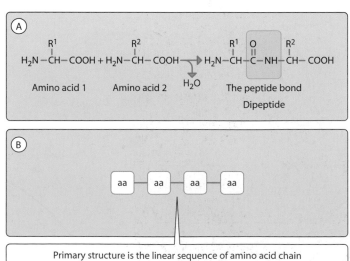

Primary structure is the linear sequence of amino acid chain

Fig. 3.16.2 The peptide bond links amino acids in a chain.

Table 3.16.1 THE AMINO ACIDS

Name	Symbol	Number of carbons	Comment
Glycine	Gly G	2	Hydrophobic
Alanine	Ala A	3	Hydrophobic
Valine	Val V	5	Hydrophobic, branched chain
Leucine	Leu L	6	Hydrophobic, branched chain
Isoleucine	Ile I	6	Hydrophobic, branched chain
Methionine	Met M	5	Hydrophobic, contains sulfur
Proline	Pro P	5	Hydrophobic, rigid planar structure
Cysteine	Cys C	3	Contains sulphydryl group, disulfide forming
Phenylalanine	Phe F	9	Hydrophobic, aromatic
Tyrosine	Tyr Y	10	Hydrophobic, aromatic
Tryptophan	Trp W	11	Hydrophobic, aromatic
Arginine	Arg R	6	Basic, protonated at neutral pH
Lysine	Lys K	6	Basic, protonated at neutral pH
Histidine	His H	6	Acidic or uncharged at neutral pH
Aspartate	Asp D	4	Dicarboxylic acid, deprotonated at neutral pH
Asparagine	Asn N	4	Amide derivative of aspartate, uncharged, participates in hydrogen bonding
Glutamate	Glu E	5	Dicarboxylic acid, deprotonated at neutral pH
Glutamine	Gln Q	5	Amide derivative of glutamate, uncharged, participates in hydrogen bonding
Serine	Ser S	3	Polar, hydroxyl groups participate in hydrogen bonding
Threonine	Thr T	4	Polar, hydroxyl groups participate in hydrogen bonding

The peptide bond

The peptide bond forms between the carboxyl group of one amino acid and the amino group of another. It is a covalent bond that forms the backbone of primary structure of the proteins (Fig. 3.16.2). There is no limitation on the length of an amino acid polymer. Each polymer will have an amino-terminus and a carboxy-terminus with a linear sequence of amino acids between. This is the *primary sequence* (see Ch. 18). Proteins with a molecular mass below 10 000 are called *polypeptides.*

17. Amino acids II

Questions

- Name three polar amino acids; how would they behave as part of a folding protein molecule?
- Which amino acid imparts rigidity on a polypeptide chain?
- Which amino acids contribute to the formation of hydrogen bonds?

Amino acids differ in their size, polarity and charge. Those with non-polar and aliphatic chains are glycine, alanine, valine, leucine, isoleucine and methionine (Fig. 3.17.1). In proteins they cluster in the interior of molecules, avoiding contact with water.

Aromatic amino acids are phenylalanine, tyrosine and tryptophan (Fig. 3.17.2). They are rather hydrophobic, although the presence of a hydroxyl group in tyrosine increases its polarity.

Amino acids with polar but uncharged groups are serine, threonine, cysteine, proline asparagine and glutamine (Fig. 3.17.3). They can form hydrogen bonds, which maintain secondary and tertiary structure of proteins.

Amino acids with positively charged groups (basic) are lysine, arginine and histidine and those with negatively charged groups (acidic) are aspartate and glutamate (Fig. 3.17.4). These charged amino acids contribute to the formation of weak bonds known as salt bridges.

The structure of an amino acid may be flexible or rigid. Proline, being a ring structure, is rigid and introduces rigidity into polypeptide chains. Methionine and cysteine contain sulphur. In methionine, a sulphur atom is contained in a thioether group, whereas in cysteine it is a thiol group, which can form strong disulphide bridges within or between protein chains.

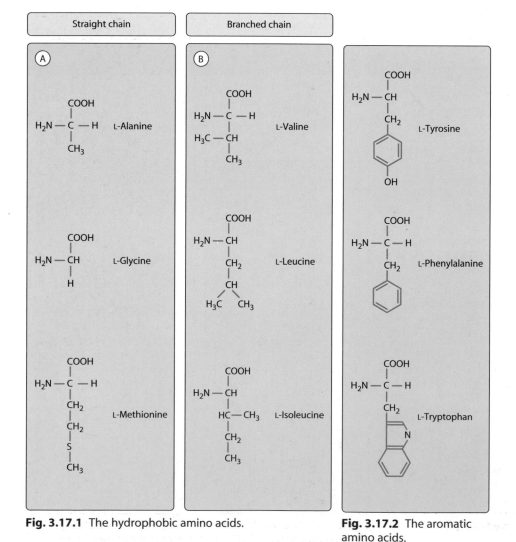

Fig. 3.17.1 The hydrophobic amino acids.

Fig. 3.17.2 The aromatic amino acids.

Note that there are two amide derivatives of amino acids: **glutamine** derived from glutamic acid, and **asparagine** derived from the aspartic acid. They contain an additional amino group and both serve as vehicles for nitrogen transport between organs.

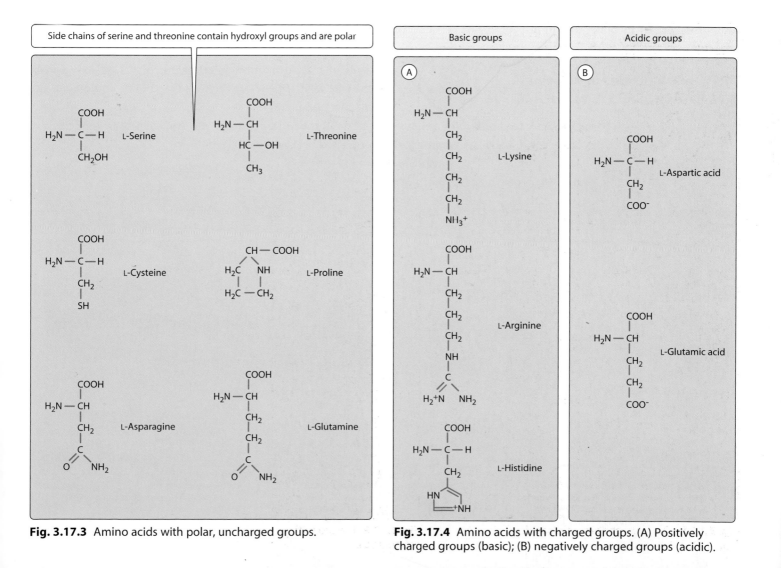

Fig. 3.17.3 Amino acids with polar, uncharged groups.

Fig. 3.17.4 Amino acids with charged groups. (A) Positively charged groups (basic); (B) negatively charged groups (acidic).

18. Proteins

Questions
- What is an example of the control of protein function by proteolytic cleavage?
- How does feedback inhibition occur?
- Which structural characteristics determine the interactions of proteins with other molecules?

The structure and function of proteins is central to biochemistry. Proteins are the expression of heredity because the information on amino acid sequence in proteins is encoded in the DNA. The catalytic proteins (enzymes) create a framework that allows every other aspect of metabolism to take place. Proteins regulate cell division and growth and provide defence against pathogens. Most of the regulatory and signalling molecules are proteins.

The number of proteins present in the body changes constantly as a result of the induction and repression of genes. The **proteome** (analogously to genome) is a sum of all the proteins in the body. The mapping of the proteome can be achieved using high-throughput technologies such as microarray chips.

Metabolic functions of proteins

Proteins perform a wide range of metabolic functions:

- structural: cell and tissue structure (e.g. collagen), architecture on which reactions can occur (e.g. ribosomal proteins)
- catalytic: enzymes
- energy production and transfer: formation of high-energy phosphate bonds and acting as molecular motors (e.g. actin and myosin in muscle contraction and ciliary movement)
- regulatory: hormones, signalling molecules (e.g. G-proteins), DNA transcription (transcription factors), phosphorylation reactions (kinases and phosphatases)
- transport, e.g. haemoglobin, ferritin, thyroid-binding globulin, transferrin
- membrane structures: channels and pores, hormone receptors, pumps, carrier proteins
- immune system, e.g. antibodies.

■ PROTEIN STRUCTURE

The **primary structure** of a protein is the sequence of amino acids joined by strong, covalent peptide bonds: –NH–CO–NH (Ch. 16). There is no limit on the potential length of the amino acid chain.

The **secondary structure** is the folding of the string of amino acids. It may form either spiral helices or flat or wavy sheets; they are held together by the hydrogen bonds and other weak interactions.

The **tertiary structure** is the way helices and sheets are organized in space.

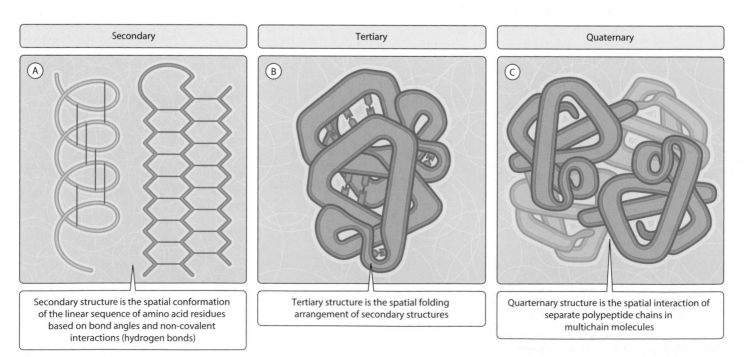

Secondary	Tertiary	Quaternary
A	B	C
Secondary structure is the spatial conformation of the linear sequence of amino acid residues based on bond angles and non-covalent interactions (hydrogen bonds)	Tertiary structure is the spatial folding arrangement of secondary structures	Quarternary structure is the spatial interaction of separate polypeptide chains in multichain molecules

Fig. 3.18.1 Protein structure.

The **quaternary structure** is the shape of multisubunit proteins. This includes supramolecular forms of proteins such as dimers, large aggregates or protein–DNA complexes.

The proper folding of proteins is of paramount importance; a special class of molecules called **chaperones** assist in this, and also unfold misfolded proteins.

Amino acid sequence determines the tridimensional structure of proteins

The primary structure of a peptide determines its secondary and tertiary structure. Thus it is the sequence of amino acids and the nature of their side chains that determines the spatial structure of the resulting protein molecule. The bonds present in a protein molecule (Fig. 3.15.3) are covalent bonds, disulphide bridges, hydrogen bonds and van der Waals forces.

Protein molecules tend to acquire the most thermodynamically stable conformation, the **native state**. Many proteins contain components such as metal ions and prosthetic groups. Protein folding is also influenced by ligands such as coenzymes or substrates, and by the interaction with allosteric effectors.

The three-dimensional structure and folding pattern are also dependent on the nature of solvent and on pH and temperature. Denaturation is the complete unfolding of a protein, which still maintains its primary structure.

Protein interactions

The hydrogen-bonding potential, charge distribution and the nature and area of the accessible surface determine the interactions of proteins with other molecules such as with carbohydrates to form glycoproteins, with fats to form lipoproteins and with DNA to form both transitory and stable complexes.

Mechanisms that control protein activity

Catalytic or signalling properties can be modified by several mechanisms.

Proteolytic cleavage. This may be a way of activating molecules before secretion (e.g. the split of proinsulin into insulin and C-peptide) or of avoiding activity in unwanted locations (e.g. secreting proteolytic enzymes in an inactive form, such as trypsinogen, to avoid autodigestion of tissue).

Reversible dimerization. Control of activity through the polymerization of two similar molecules, e.g. membrane phospholipase A.

Covalent modification. The phosphorylation/dephosphorylation mechanism is the most common way of regulating enzymes and pathways. Phosphorylation of enzyme molecules at serine, threonine or tyrosine residues is common in cellular signalling cascades.

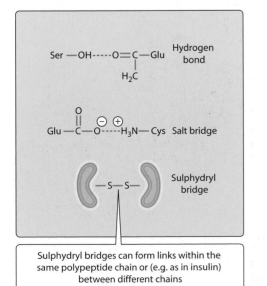

Sulphydryl bridges can form links within the same polypeptide chain or (e.g. as in insulin) between different chains

Fig. 3.18.2 Examples of covalent and non-covalent bonds within protein molecules.

19. Simple and complex carbohydrates

Questions
- What is the structural basis for carbohydrate diversity?
- Which chemical bonds are important in polymerization of carbohydrates?
- What is the biological importance of carbohydrates linked to proteins?

Carbohydrates are the key metabolic fuel. They are also structural components of cells, particularly when linked to proteins or lipids. Glycolipids and glycoproteins are fundamental for such functions as cell–cell recognition.

Carbohydrates: molecules with 'hidden' diversity

Diversity of carbohydrates is achieved by changes in the spatial structure, such as differences in positioning of hydroxyl residues and hydrogen ions around carbon atoms, and the many ways of forming polymers.

In the structure of a sugar, carbon-1 is anomeric. Configuration of other atoms around this carbon gives rise to two series of

stereoisomers, α and β (Fig. 3.19.1). Most biologically important sugars belong to the α-series. There also are optical isomers, which rotate the plane of polarized light either to the right (they are designated +) or to the left (−). The biologically important sugars are dextrorotatory.

In solution, carbohydrates form either linear or ring structures known as furanose and pyranose: 99% glucose in a solution is in the form of pyranose. Some sugars possess aldehyde groups (**aldoses**); others have keto groups (**ketoses**). Glucose is an aldose and fructose is a ketose (Fig. 3.19.1). The most important aldoses and ketoses are illustrated in Figure 3.19.2.

Sugars that differ in configuration of carbons other than the anomeric carbon are **epimers**. Glucose, mannose and galactose differ with respect to the configuration around carbon-2 (mannose) or carbon-4 (galactose) (Fig. 3.19.3).

Polymeric forms of carbohydrates
Carbohydrates form oligomers and polymers. The simplest units, which cannot be hydrolysed any further, are **monosaccharides**. **Disaccharides** contain two monosacharide units, **oligosaccharides** 2–10 units and **polysaccharides** more than 10 units.

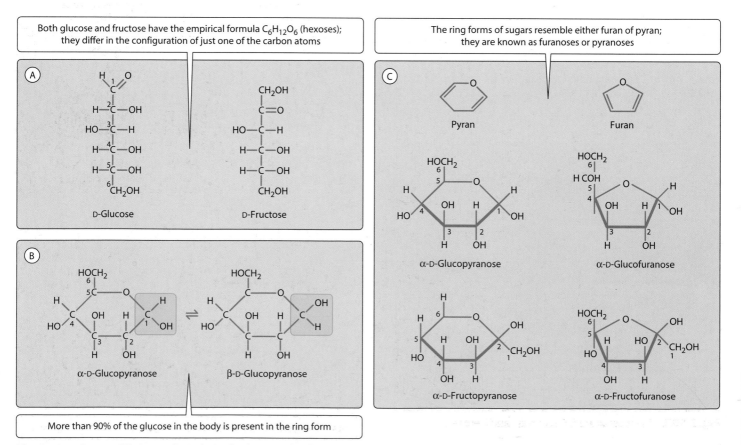

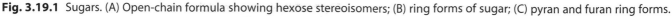

Fig. 3.19.1 Sugars. (A) Open-chain formula showing hexose stereoisomers; (B) ring forms of sugar; (C) pyran and furan ring forms.

The way sugars form polymers is an important source of carbohydrate diversity. The important bond here is the **glycosidic bond** (Fig. 3.19.4): it results from condensation of hydroxyl group of the anomeric carbon of a carbohydrate and either a sugar (*O*-glycoside) or an amine (*N*-glycoside) The *N*-glycosidic bonds are common between nucleotides (e.g. adenine) and sugars such as ribose or deoxyribose (Ch. 45). Amino sugars include D-glucosamine, galactosamine and mannosamine. *N*-Acetyl derivatives of carbohydrates are present in glycoproteins.

Disaccharides are two monosaccharides linked by an *O*-glycosidic bond. Examples are maltose, sucrose and lactose.

The most important **polysaccharides** are starch, glucogen and cellulose.

Starch. This plant polysaccharide starch has glycosidic bonds linking C1 to C4 and is the main component of potatoes cereals and legumes.

Glycogen. This animal storage carbohydrate is structurally similar to starch: it has chains of 12–14 glucose residues linked by 1–4 glycosidic bonds; branches form by 1–6 bonds.

Cellulose. The plant polymer cellulose has glucose residues linked by β(1–4) bond.

Carbohydrates attached to proteins

Carbohydrates linked to proteins stabilize structure and sometimes protect them from degradation; they also enhance their solubility. Because of their diversity, they (similarly to glycolipids) serve as cellular recognition signals.

Glycoproteins are hybrids of proteins and carbohydrates and are essential surface components of biological membranes. Glycosylated residues are also important in collagen. Oligosaccharides form parts of cellular receptors. Glycoproteins contain sialic acids, which are *N*- or *O*-acyl derivatives of neuraminic acid (a 9-carbon carbohydrate derived from mannosamine and pyruvate).

Glycosaminoglycans (mucopolysaccharides) such as hyaluronic acid are the carbohydrate parts of proteoglycans. They are highly polar, which facilitates hydration and keeps the proteins unfolded. Glycosaminoglycans and proteoglycans are the main components of the extracellular matrix.

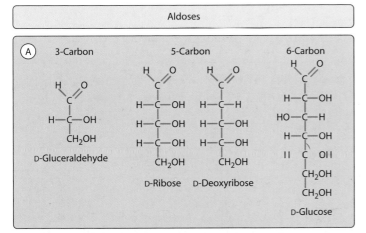

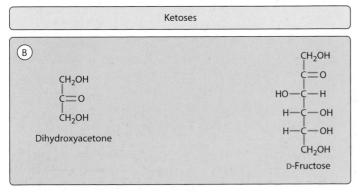

Fig. 3.19.2 The most important aldoses and ketoses.

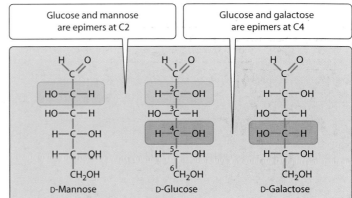

Fig. 3.19.3 The epimers.

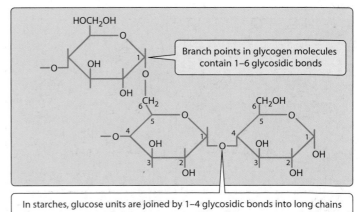

Fig. 3.19.4 The *O*-glycosidic bond.

20. Simple and complex lipids

Questions
- What is the structure of neutral fats?
- What is meant by saying that membrane lipids are amphipathic?
- Where does diacylglycerol fit into hormonal signalling cascades?

Lipids are important as

- High-energy storage fuel
- source of heat: brown fat is a specialized heat-producing tissue
- structural molecules, e.g. in biological membranes
- signalling species, e.g. the phosphoinositol system
- insulation: both thermal and electrical (myelin).

Structure of lipids

The simplest lipids are the fatty acids: hydrophobic molecules of 4–36 carbon length, some with variable numbers of double bonds. The chain length and the degree of saturation of the hydrocarbon chain determine the degree of their fluidity. Fatty acids with no double bonds are **saturated**. The most important are palmitic and the stearic acids. Those with one double bond are **monounsaturated**, and those with multiple double bonds are **polyunsaturated** (Fig. 3.20.1). The *cis*-type double bond introduces a kink to the structure that interferes with the packing of these molecules in membranes, increasing membrane fluidity. This also lowers their melting point.

Description of a fatty acid includes the number of carbons in the molecule and the number and position of its double bonds. The carboxyl (end) carbon is designated C1. The next carbon from the carboxyl end is known as the α-carbon. The last one (the 'front-end' or the 'methyl end' carbon) is known as the omega (ω) carbon. Polyunsaturated fatty acids are classed by the place of the first double bond, counting from the omega end of the molecule: thus we have ω-6 and ω-3 fatty acids. The designation gives the number of carbon atoms and the number and position of double bonds: so 18:2, Δ9,12 indicates 18 carbon atoms, 2 double bonds with the double bonds at positions 9 and 12 counting from the omega end.

Fatty acids are ionized at physiological pH and are transported in plasma bound to albumin. Some fatty acids cannot be synthesized in the body; these are known as the **essential fatty acids**. They are

- linoleic acid, an ω-6 acid (18:2, Δ9,12), which is the precursor of arachidonic acid
- linoleic acid, an ω-6 fatty acid (18:3, Δ9,12,15)

Neutral fats

Neutral fats are **triacylglycerols**, also known as triglycerides (Fig. 3.20.2). Glycerol 3-phosphate used in the synthesis of triacylglycerols derives from either the phosphorylation of glycerol in the liver by glycerol kinase, or from the reduction

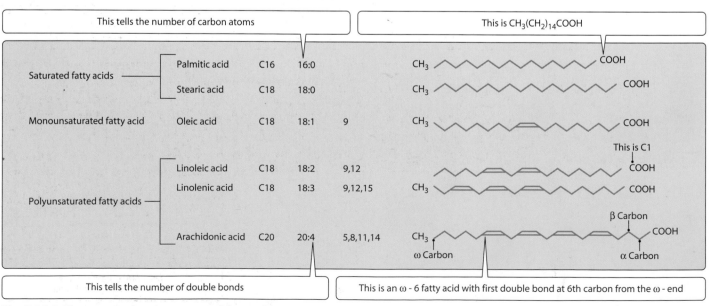

Fig. 3.20.1 The saturated and unsaturated fatty acids.

of the glycolytic intermediate dihydroxyacetone phosphate. Triacylglycerols are the main form of storage fat in tissues, particularly in the adipose tissue. Glycerol can be esterified on its three carbons with different fatty acids.

Complex lipids

Complex lipids are derivatives of diacylphosphoglycerol or another long-chain amino alcohol, **sphingosine**. The core of complex lipid molecule is the **phosphatide** (phosphoglyceride or phosphoglycerol); this is a phosphorylated diacylglycerol. Phosphatides can be esterified by other alcohols such as serine or inositol. Such **phospholipids** are key components of biological membranes (Fig. 3.20.2).

Nomenclature of complex lipids

Phospholipids are named by reference to the core backbone.

The **glycerophospholipids** have a glycerol base and may contain phosphatidylcholine, phosphatidylethanolamine or phos-phoinositol as their polar group. They contain a saturated fatty acid (C16, C18) at carbon-1 and an unsaturated fatty acid at carbon-2.

The **sphingolipids ceramides** contain sphingosine have just one acyl residue linked through the amide bond and one hydroxyl residue. In sphingomyelin, a phosphatidyl choline is joined to the hydroxyl group of sphingosine.

The **glycolipids** contain glucose and **gangliosides** possess several residues of sialic acid.

Inborn errors of lipid metabolism

Inborn errors in the metabolism of complex lipids are a cause for a range of mostly very rare diseases (e.g. the sphingolipodoses). The discussion of these disorders is beyond the scope of this book and the reader is referred to more detailed textbooks of biochemistry and clinical chemistry.

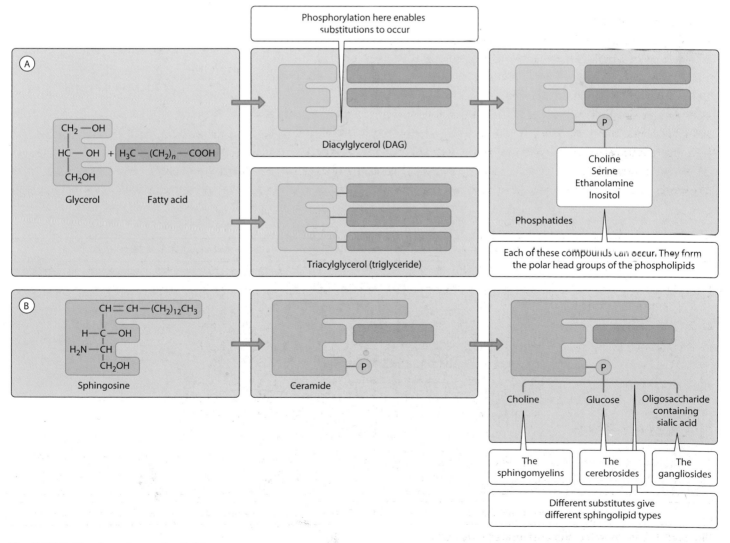

Fig. 3.20.2 Simple and complex lipids.

21. Digestion of carbohydrates, fats and proteins

Questions

- What is the endocrine function of the gastrointestinal tract?
- Why does vomiting lead to metabolic alkalosis?
- What is the difference between the action of phospholipase and that of the pancreatic lipase?

All nutrients enter the body through the gastrointestinal (GI) tract (Fig. 3.21.1). The initial stages of digestion (chewing and digestion of carbohydrates by salivary amylase) take place in the mouth; the second stage in the stomach and duodenum. The liver secretes bile and the pancreas secretes digestive enzymes. The ileum, where most digestion occurs, has a brush border that contains enzymes to carry out the final digestion of proteins, carbohydrates and fats.

The GI tract is an active endocrine organ. The stomach secretes **gastrin**, which stimulates the secretion of the hydrochloric acid by the parietal cells. The pancreas produces **secretin** and **cholecystokinin–pancreozymin**, which stimulates secretion of trypsinogen, chymotrypsinogen and procarboxypeptidases A and B. The small intestine secretes **serotonin** and **vasoactive intestinal polypeptide** (VIP). Digestion is also under neural (neurotransmitter) control: acetylcholine affects salivary, gastric, pancreatic and intestinal secretion, and histamine interacts with stomach H_2 receptors.

Carbohydrates

Polysaccharides are first digested by salivary and pancreatic **amylase**, yielding maltose, maltotriose and limit dextrins (short molecules linked by 1–6 bonds) (Fig. 3.21.2). Further digestion takes place in the ileum. Oligosaccharidases (e.g. α-glucosidase) digest complex carbohydrates. **Maltase, sucrase/isomaltase** and **lactase** in the brush border digest disaccharides into monosaccharides: mainly D-glucose, D-galactose and D-fructose.

The movement of glucose across membranes involves **glucose transporters**: Na^+-coupled monosaccharide transporters (SGLT) and the Na^+-independent monosaccharide transport facilitators (GLUT). SGLT is found on the luminal surface and GLUT2 on the contralateral membrane.

Carbohydrates not digested by the GI enzymes pass into the ileum where they can still be partially digested by bacteria, forming, among other products, hydrogen and methane gas.

Lipids

Approximately 90% of ingested lipids are triacylglycerols. Others are cholesterol, cholesteryl esters, phospholipids and free fatty acids. The stomach contains acid-stable **lipase**, which produces fatty acids and diacylglycerols. Lipids are solubilized by the bile, which acts as a detergent and emulsifies lipids into micelles (Fig. 3.21.3).

Triacylglycerols are hydrolysed by pancreatic lipase (which needs colipase for activity) (Fig. 3.18.4). Pancreatic lipid esterase acts on cholesteryl esters and monoglycerides. Phospholipids are digested by phospholipase A_2. Next, monoglycerides are taken up

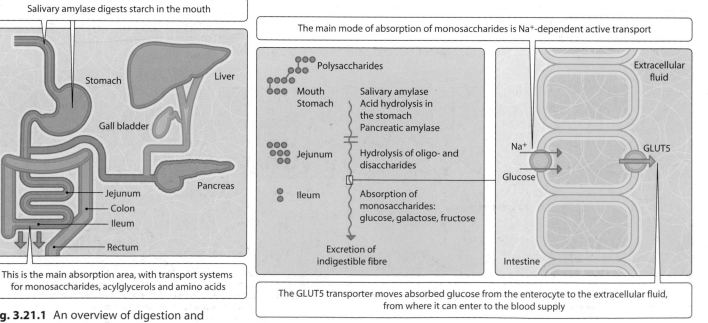

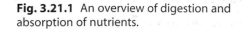

Fig. 3.21.1 An overview of digestion and absorption of nutrients.

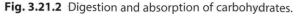

Fig. 3.21.2 Digestion and absorption of carbohydrates.

by enterocytes, which actively resynthesize triacylglycerols and assemble **chylomicrons.** Chylomicrons leave enterocytes by exocytosis and reach the circulation through the lymph. Medium-length fatty acids (C6–C10) pass directly into portal blood.

Proteins

Ingested proteins are first denatured by hydrochloric acid secreted by the parietal cells of the stomach (Fig. 3.21.4). Pancreatic juice contains **pepsinogen** (a **zymogen**) that is autoactivated by **pepsin** in the intestine. The pancreas also secretes bicarbonate, which increases the pH of the duodenum. The other major peptidases are **trypsin** (secreted as trypsinogen and converted to trypsin by intestinal enteropeptidase), **chymotrypsin** (secreted as chymotrypsinogen) and **carboxypeptidases A and B** (also secreted as procarboxypeptidases).

MALABSORPTION SYNDROMES

Congenital defects in the sugar transporters lead to various disorders, for example the glucose–galactose malabsorption syndrome (SGLT1) and Fanconi–Bickel syndrome (GLUT2).

Gastrointestinal disorders associated with malabsorption, such as Crohn's disease or ulcerative colitis, may lead to nutritional deficiencies and to profound water and electrolyte disorders. Patients, particularly after surgical intervention, may require long-term intravenous nutrition.

Further digestion takes place in the ileum by brush border carboxypeptidases and aminopeptidases and also by **alkaline phosphatase**, which digests organic phosphates. The resulting free amino acids are absorbed into the enterocytes by specific transport systems.

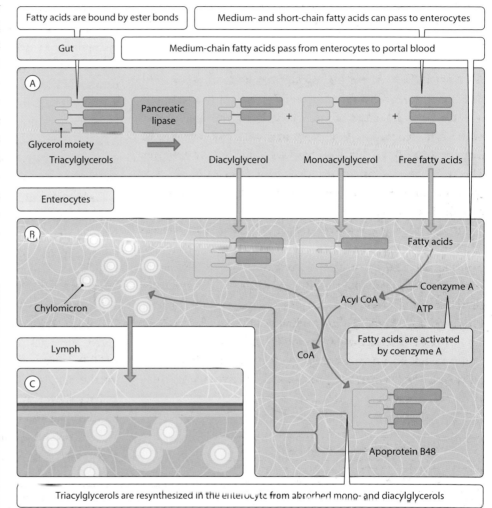

Fig. 3.21.4 Metabolism of triacylglycerols.

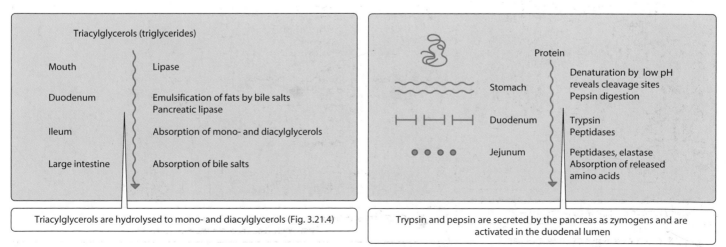

Fig. 3.21.3 Digestion and absorption of fats.

Fig. 3.21.5 Digestion and absorption of proteins.

22. Lipoproteins

Questions
- What are lipoprotein remnants?
- What are the roles of the different lipoprotein classes?

Fatty acids are either acquired with the diet or synthesized in the liver. They are either oxidized or are converted to triacylglycerols in the liver and the triacylglycerols are transported to their main storage site, the adipose tissue. Free fatty acids travel in blood bound to serum albumin, but triacylglycerols are transported between organs as components of particles known as lipoproteins.

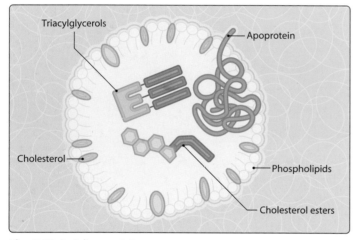

Fig. 3.22.1 A lipoprotein.

The lipoproteins

Lipoproteins are lipidated protein molecules: in other words, heterogeneous lipid droplets assembled on protein particles in the liver or intestine (Fig. 3.22.1). Their component proteins are called apolipoproteins. During lipoprotein assembly, the hydrophilic components such as cholesterol and phospholipid remain on the outer surface, and the hydrophobic components such as cholesteryl esters and, particularly, triacylglycerols locate in the core of the particles. The apolipoproteins drive the metabolism of these particles by binding to cellular membrane receptors. Importantly, lipoprotein lipids also contain other dissolved molecules such as vitamins A and E. Vitamin E plays an important role protecting lipids from oxidation.

Lipoproteins differ in size and composition. They are classified on the basis of their density in separations performed using ultracentrifugation or electrophoresis. The different classes of lipoprotein are:

- chylomicrons
- very low density lipoproteins (VLDL)
- intermediate density lipoproteins (IDL; also known as remnant particles)
- low density lipoproteins (LDL)
- high density lipoproteins (HDL).

Different types of lipoprotein contain specific apoproteins (e.g. ApoE in very low density lipoproteins). The different classes of

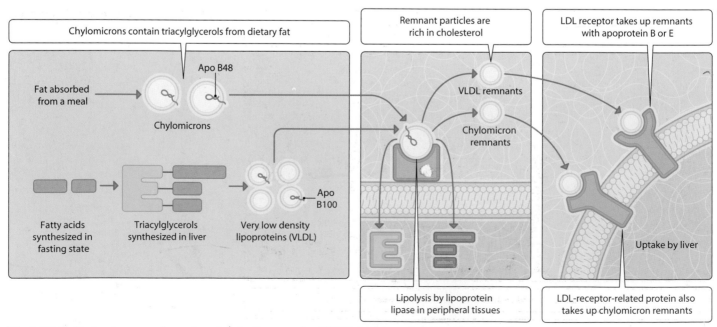

Fig. 3.22.2 Chylomicrons and very low density lipoproteins (VLDL) transport fuel to tissues.

lipoprotein have specific functions (Table 3.22.1 and Fig. 3.22.2). The synthesis, metabolism and elimination of a lipoprotein is illustrated in Fig. 3.22.3. Chapter 23 describes the role of lipoproteins in transporting lipids between organs.

Fatty acid interactions with protein

Fatty acids, particularly the polyunsaturated fatty acids, are ligands for transcription factors, which regulate genes involved in the energy metabolism. For example, they play an important role in the regulation of insulin sensitivity. They upregulate genes involved in lipid oxidation in the liver and skeletal muscle and downregulate genes involved in lipogenesis in the liver and in the adipose tissue. They also induce the expression of the mitochondrial uncoupling protein-2 and uncoupling protein-3 in the skeletal muscle, and thus increase thermogenesis.

Table 3.22.1 MAJOR FUNCTIONS OF LIPOPROTEINS

Lipoprotein	Functions
VLDL	Transport of triacylglycerols from liver to adipose tissue
LDL	High cholesteryl ester content; delivers cholesterol to the liver and extrahepatic tissues
HDL	Removal of cholesterol from cells
Chylomicrons	Transport of triacylglycerols from GI tract

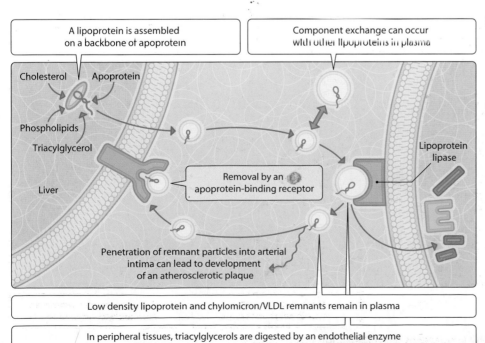

Fig. 3.22.3 Natural history of a lipoprotein.

A lipoprotein is assembled on a backbone of apoprotein

Component exchange can occur with other lipoproteins in plasma

Cholesterol

Apoprotein

Phospholipids

Triacylglycerol

Liver

Lipoprotein lipase

Removal by an apoprotein-binding receptor

Penetration of remnant particles into arterial intima can lead to development of an atherosclerotic plaque

Low density lipoprotein and chylomicron/VLDL remnants remain in plasma

In peripheral tissues, triacylglycerols are digested by an endothelial enzyme

23. Lipoproteins and the transport of lipids

Questions
- How does highly density lipoprotein 'return' cholesterol to the liver?
- Which lipoprotein particles are atherogenic?
- What does the measurement of serum total cholesterol reflect?

The inter-organ transport of lipids

Lipoproteins form a transport system that distributes triacylglycerols from the liver and intestine mainly to the adipose tissue and muscle (see Fig. 3.22.2). In this sense, the lipoprotein transport pathway involving chylomicrons, VLDL and remnant particles is part of the body energy metabolism.

If the smaller lipoproteins (the remnants and LDL) are present in excess in plasma, they may deposit in the arterial walls; the lipids that they carry can then become centres of atherosclerotic plaques (Fig. 3.23.1). This is the basis of the lipid hypothesis of **atherosclerosis** (see Ch. 60). Clearly, atherosclerosis depends on the burden placed on the lipid transport system.

Pathways of lipid transport

After a fat-containing meal, chylomicrons transport triacylglycerols from the intestine to the liver and to peripheral tissues. Chylomicron remnants return to the liver.

In the fasting state, the liver still sends a limited amount of lipids to the periphery by assembling the triacylglycerol-rich VLDL with a backbone of apoprotein B100 (instead of apoB48 in chylomicrons) (Fig. 3.23.1). The VLDL–IDL–LDL pathway transports lipids to the periphery and returns most of cholesterol back to the liver through the LDL receptor.

In the peripheral tissues, the triacylglycerols (both in chylomicrons and VLDL) undergo partial hydrolysis (lipolysis) by the enzyme **lipoprotein lipase**. As a result, glycerol is released, and fatty acids are taken up by cells. What remains are lipoproteins poorer in triacylglycerols, and now relatively rich in cholesterol: these are called chylomicron remnants and VLDL remnants. The remnants are either taken up by the LDL receptor (chylomicron remnants bind also to the LDL-receptor-related protein), mostly in the liver but also in the peripheral tissues, or are further hydrolysed by hepatic lipase, yielding a still smaller particle, the LDL. LDL particles are also poor in triacylglycerols and rich in cholesterol and, similarly to the remnant particles, are taken up by the cellular LDL receptor. The LDL are small enough to penetrate arterial endothelium, particularly if it is functionally damaged: they are the main lipoprotein seen in the atherosclerotic plaques. Lowering LDL concentration in plasma is one of the pillars of cardiovascular prevention.

The LDL can be pictured as an 'overflow lipoprotein' generated by fuel metabolism: when the fuel transport pathway is for any

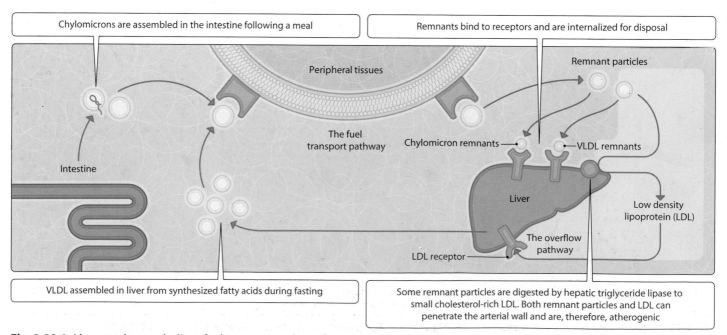

Chylomicrons are assembled in the intestine following a meal

Remnants bind to receptors and are internalized for disposal

Peripheral tissues

Remnant particles

The fuel transport pathway

Chylomicron remnants

VLDL remnants

Intestine

Liver

Low density lipoprotein (LDL)

The overflow pathway

LDL receptor

VLDL assembled in liver from synthesized fatty acids during fasting

Some remnant particles are digested by hepatic triglyceride lipase to small cholesterol-rich LDL. Both remnant particles and LDL can penetrate the arterial wall and are, therefore, atherogenic

Fig. 3.23.1 Lipoprotein metabolism: fuel transport and overflow pathways.

University Hospitals of Derby & Burton
NHS Foundation Trust
01332 788146

Mail: uhdb.library@nhs.net

Self Service Receipt for Borrowing

Patron: Lynsey Harrower

Title: Flesh and bones of metabolism
Item: 1005025443
Due Back: 28/01/2020

Title: Down syndrome : the facts
Item: B14148
Due Back: 28/01/2020

Total Borrowing: 2
03/12/2019 12:27:07

Thank you and see you soon

reason overloaded, more LDL arises from remnant particles (Fig. 3.23.1).

Reverse cholesterol transport

The other important component of the lipid transport system is so-called reverse cholesterol transport: transport of cholesterol from peripheral tissues to the liver for reutilization (Fig. 3.23.2). The central particle in the so-called reverse cholesterol transport is HDL. Analogously to VLDL being constructed on the backbone of apoB, HDL is assembled in the liver and intestine by the lipidation of the lipid-poor apoAI. Cholesterol is transferred from cells to apoAI by way of the membrane transporter called ABCA1. The resulting particle 'matures' when its cholesterol is esterified by **lecithin–cholesterol acyltransferase** (LCAT). At this stage, HDL transfers some cholesteryl esters to triacylglycerol-rich lipoproteins (VLDL or IDL) in exchange for triacylglycerols. When the mature HDL reaches the liver, cholesteryl esters are transferred to the hepatocyte by the scavenger receptor SR-B1. Remaining delipidated apoprotein re-enters the transport cycle. The measurements of plasma cholesterol, LDL-cholesterol, plasma triglycerols and HDL-cholesterol constitute the **lipid profile** routinely measured in clinical laboratories.

INBORN ERRORS OF LIPOPROTEIN METABOLISM

Inborn errors in the metabolism of lipoproteins are a cause for a range of disorders, the most common being the familial hypercholesterolaemia associated with mutations in the gene for the LDL receptor. Lipoprotein disorders associated with hypercholesterolaemia and combined dyslipidaemia tend to be associated with premature atherosclerosis, and those leading to isolated severe hypertriglyceridaemia are associated with pancreatitis.

High cholesterol concentration is not the only lipid pattern associated with an increased cardiovascular risk. Low HDL-cholesterol (usually associated with an increased ratio of total cholesterol to HDL-cholesterol) is also an important risk factor.

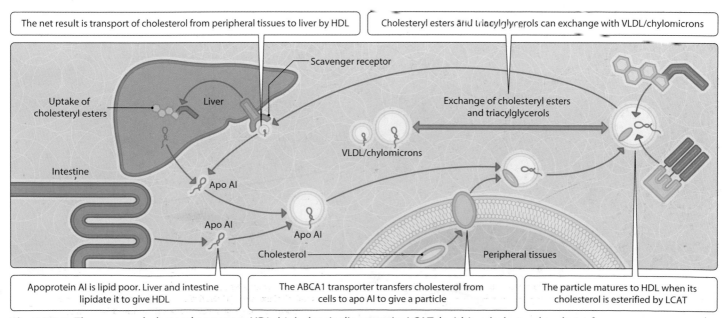

The net result is transport of cholesterol from peripheral tissues to liver by HDL

Cholesteryl esters and triacylglycerols can exchange with VLDL/chylomicrons

Scavenger receptor

Uptake of cholesteryl esters

Liver

Exchange of cholesteryl esters and triacylglycerols

VLDL/chylomicrons

Intestine

Apo AI

Apo AI

Apo AI

Cholesterol

Peripheral tissues

Apoprotein AI is lipid poor. Liver and intestine lipidate it to give HDL

The ABCA1 transporter transfers cholesterol from cells to apo AI to give a particle

The particle matures to HDL when its cholesterol is esterified by LCAT

Fig. 3.23.2 The reverse cholesterol transport. HDL, high density lipoprotein; LCAT, lecithin–cholesterol acyltransferase.

24. Glycolysis: overview

Questions
- What tissues depend on glycolysis for energy?
- What happens to pyruvate in exercising muscle?

The role of glycolysis

Glycolysis is the main pathway of glucose metabolism in the cell. It can operate in both the presence and the absence of O_2 and, therefore, is fundamentally important for the exercising muscle and for erythrocytes (which do not possess mitochondria). The energy yield of anaerobic glycolysis, however, is much lower than that of aerobic metabolism of glucose.

In the hypoxic conditions, glycolysis yields lactate (Fig. 3.24.1). In the presence of O_2, the final metabolite is pyruvate (Fig. 3.24.2). Pyruvate feeds into the Krebs cycle through the reaction catalysed by **pyruvate dehydrogenase** (PDH). Glycolysis occurs in the cytoplasm.

Anaerobic and aerobic pyruvate metabolism

Anaerobic lactate production. In anaerobic conditions, pyruvate undergoes reduction by NADH to lactate, catalysed by

[handwritten annotation: builds up in tissue and blood → lactic acidosis in prolonged periods of hypoxia]

lactate dehydrogenase. This reaction regenerates the NAD^+ that had been used in the glyceraldehyde-3-phosphate dehydrogenase reaction, allowing anaerobic glycolysis to continue without the need for NAD^+ regeneration in the mitochondria. In the liver, **pyruvate kinase**, which converts phosphoenolpyruvate to pyruvate, is inhibited by glucagon. In both muscle and liver it is stimulated by F1,6BP (this is known as feed-forward stimulation).

Aerobic acetyl-CoA production. When O_2 is available, PDH converts pyruvate into acetyl-CoA, a metabolite of the Krebs cycle. PDH is another enzyme subject to multiple controls.

The important branch points of glycolysis

The major branch points are shown in Figure 3.24.1:

- glycogenogenesis from glucose 6-phosphate
- pentose phosphate pathway from glucose 6-phosphate
- glycerol 3-phosphate synthesis from dihydroxyacetone phosphate.

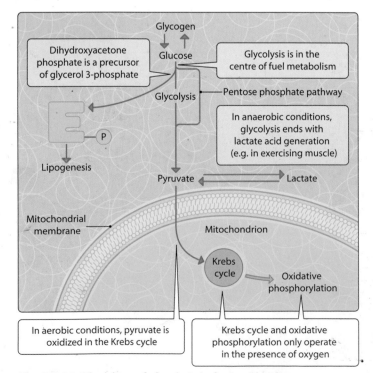

Fig. 3.24.1 The place of glycolysis in fuel metabolism.

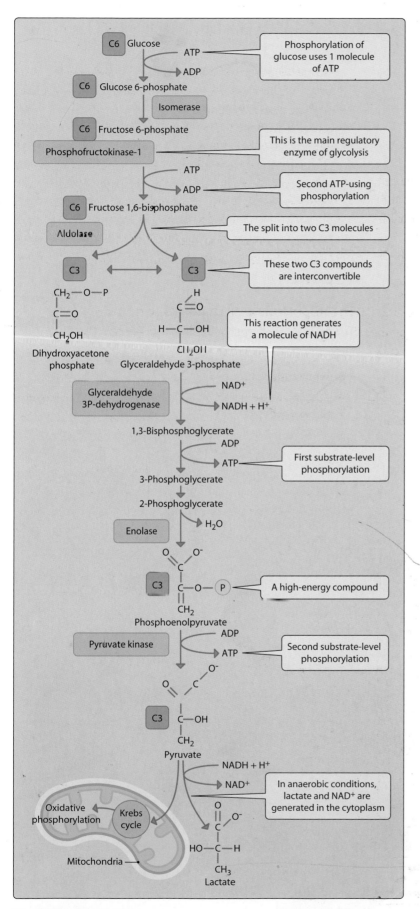

Fig. 3.24.2 Glycolysis.

25. Glycolysis: energy consumption and production

Questions
- The regulation of hexokinase by glucose differs in liver and muscle; what are the metabolic consequences of this?
- What are the relationships between phosphofructokinase-1 and phosphofructokinase-2?
- What substrate-level phosphorylations occur in glycolysis?

It is convenient to discuss glycolysis by dividing it into energy-consuming and energy-yielding stages.

Energy-consuming stage of glycolysis
Once glucose has entered the cell, it is phosphorylated by **hexokinase** (or its isoenzyme **glucokinase** in the liver and in the beta-cells of the pancreas) (see Fig. 3.24.2). Both enzymes phosphorylate glucose using ATP. Glucokinase has a higher K_m than hexokinase (10 mmol/l versus 0.1 mmol/l); therefore, it is more efficient at higher glucose concentrations such as those that occur after a meal.

Muscle hexokinase, but not liver glucokinase, is inhibited by its product, glucose 6-phosphate (Glc6P); this improves the economy of use of glucose in muscle. In the liver, the enzyme phosphorylates all glucose available, and the excess is eventually converted to fat. This is how eating excess of carbohydrates leads to weight gain.

Subsequently, Glc6P is isomerized to fructose 6-phosphate (F6P) by phosphoglucomutase, and F6P is phosphorylated, again using ATP, by **phosphofructokinase-1** (PFK-1). This is the main regulatory hub of glycolysis. It is controlled by two cooperating enzymes: PFK-1 in the 'main' pathway and a bifunctional PFK-2/**fructose-2,6-phosphatase** (Fig. 3.25.1). PFK-1 is stimulated by fructose 2,6-bisphosphate (F2,6-BP), the product of the PFK-2 reaction. Both ATP and the Krebs cycle metabolite citrate inhibit PFK-1. The inhibition is relieved by 'low energy' ADP and AMP; thus glycolysis is controlled by the energy status of the cell (Fig. 3.25.2). The regulatory role of PFK-2 is discussed in more detail below.

The regulatory role of phosphofructokinase-2
The PFK-2/F2,6Pase is subject to regulation by hormone-stimulated phosphorylation involving the G-protein–cAMP–protein kinase A signalling cascade. The product of PFK-2, F2,6-BP, allosterically stimulates **fructokinase** in the 'main' glycolytic pathway (PFK-1) and inhibits the opposite reaction catalysed by **fructose-1,6,-bisphosphatase** (Fig. 3.20.2). Therefore, under the influence of F2,6-BP, glycolysis is stimulated and gluconeogenesis inhibited.

PFK-2 is controlled differently in different tissues. In heart muscle, PFK-1/F2,6Pase is regulated by epinephrine. In skeletal muscle, PFK-2 is stimulated simply by the glycolytic inter-

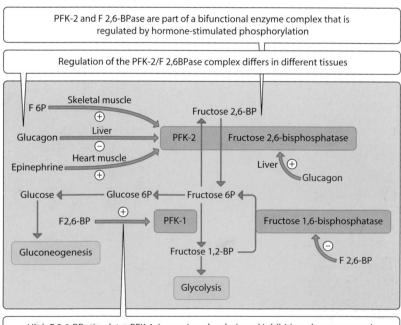

Fig. 3.25.1 Regulation of glycolysis by fructose 2,6-bisphosphate.

mediate F6P. In the liver, PFK-2 is inactivated by glucagon (inhibiting glycolysis) and F2,6Pase is activated, stimulating gluconeogenesis.

Energy-yielding stage of glycolysis

There are two substrate-level phosphorylations in glycolysis: the first is is catalysed by **phosphoglycerate kinase** and the second by **pyruvate kinase**.

The product of the PFK-1 reaction, fructose 1,6-bisphosphate (F1,6,BP), is split by aldolase into two interconvertible 3-carbon molecules: dihydroxyacetone phosphate (DHAP) and glyceraldehyde 3-phosphate (Fig. 3.20.2). DHAP serves an important intermediary in the production of glycerol 3-phosphate, a platform for triaglycerol synthesis (see p. 91).

Glyceraldehyde 3-phosphate is oxidized (its aldehyde group is converted to a carboxyl group) by glyceraldehyde-3-phosphate dehydrogenase (an enzyme using NAD$^+$) to **1,3-bisphosphoglycerate**, a high-energy compound. Phosphoglycerate kinase then transfers the high-energy phosphate group to ATP, and yields 3-phosphoglycerate. This is the first substrate-level phosphorylation in glycolysis.

The 3-phosphoglycerate is next transformed by a magnesium-dependent phosphoglycerate mutase into 2-phosphoglycerate, which, after dehydration, generates another high-energy compound, **phosphoenolpyruvate** (PEP). PEP becomes a substrate for the second substrate-level phosphorylation in glycolysis, conducted by pyruvate kinase, yielding a 3-carbon key metabolite, pyruvate.

The energy yield of glycolysis

The net energy yield of glycolysis is 2 ATP. Each 6-carbon molecule of glucose generates two interconvertible 3-carbon molecules. Therefore the two substrate-level phosphorylations yield 2 ATP per C3 moiety: 4 ATP altogether. However, 2 ATP are used at the initial stage of glycolysis to phosphorylate glucose and F6P. This decreases the net yield to 2 ATP.

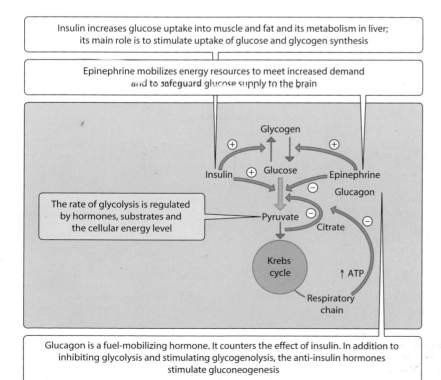

Fig. 3.25.2 The principal regulators of glycolysis.

26. Krebs cycle (tricarboxylic acid cycle) I

Questions
- Which Krebs cycle reactions yield NADH?
- Which enzyme links the glycolytic pathway to the Krebs cycle and provides acetyl-CoA?
- What is an anaplerotic reaction and what example can you give?

The Krebs cycle, also known as tricarboxylic acid cycle, is the focal point of the entire cellular metabolism (Fig. 3.26.1). It provides the majority of electrons for the mitochondrial oxidations, and a range of substrates for diverse biosynthetic reactions. It integrates carbohydrate, lipid and protein metabolism, creating a common gateway to the mitochondrial respiratory chain. In contrast to glycolysis, the cycle operates only in aerobic conditions. It oxidizes the C2 acetyl-CoA molecule, generating $NADH^+$, H^+, $FADH_2$ and CO_2.

Cellular location and metabolic role
The Krebs cycle receives metabolites from several pathways. It links directly with glycolysis and forms the second major segment of glucose metabolism. From the energetics point of view, the essence of the Krebs cycle is oxidation (electron-harvesting) reactions yielding reduced nucleotides NADH and $FADH_2$. These, in turn, become substrates for the mitochondrial electron transport chain.

Enzymes of the Krebs cycle are located in the mitochondrial matrix, except for succinate dehydrogenase (a FAD-dependent enzyme), which resides in the inner mitochondrial membrane, close to the electron transport chain. The mitochondrial location of the cycle, however, creates a transport problem; several key metabolites need to enter and exit the mitochondria, but the inner mitochondrial membrane is highly selective to molecules. Therefore, the metabolites that cannot be transported by existing transport systems need to be first converted to 'transportable' intermediates.

The entry of pyruvate into the cycle: pyruvate conversion to acetyl-CoA
The mitochondrial matrix enzyme pyruvate dehydrogenase (PDH) catalyses oxidative decarboxylation of pyruvate to acetyl-CoA (this reaction provides a key substrate for, but does not itself belong to, the Krebs cycle) (Fig. 3.26.2). Note that, similarly to the reactions in the cycle itself, the PDH reaction generates NADH:

$$pyruvate + CoA + NAD^+ \rightleftharpoons acetyl\text{-}CoA + CO_2 + NADH + H^+$$

PDH is a large multienzyme complex containing three enzymes (designated E1–E3) and involves interactions with coenzyme thiamin pyrophosphate (TPP), lipoic acid, FAD, NAD^+ and CoA.

Pyruvate first binds to TPP and is decarboxylated by the dehydrogenase E1. Oxidation to acetate takes place together with transfer to lipoamide. Next, the acetyl group is transferred from lipoamide to CoA, forming acetyl-CoA; this is catalysed by dihydrolipoyl transacetylase (enzyme E_2). The reduced lipoamide is reoxidized by dihydrolipolyl dehydrogenase, which uses FAD as a hydrogen acceptor, and from there the electrons are transferred to NAD^+.

The compact structure of the complex makes the reactions more efficient. The mechanism of action of this multienzyme complex is the same as that of the Krebs cycle α-ketoglutarate dehydrogenase and branched-chain amino acid dehydrogenase.

Regulation of pyruvate dehydrogenase complex
PDH is inhibited by its product acetyl-CoA and also by NADH (Fig. 3.21.3). It is also regulated by phosphorylation–dephosphorylation carried out by a kinase and a phosphatase.

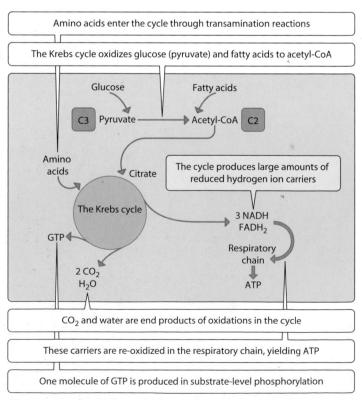

Fig. 3.26.1 The Krebs cycle integrates carbohydrate, fat and protein metabolism.

Acetyl-coenzyme A

The PDH reaction is but one source of acetyl-CoA. The other major one is the beta-oxidation of fatty acids. Several (ketogenic Ch. 40) amino acids are also catabolized to acetyl-CoA. Regard acetyl-CoA as one of the major 'common metabolic currency' compounds (see Ch. 38). The transport of acetyl-CoA to the cytosol (and other metabolic shuttles) is described in Ch. 29.

 PYRUVATE DEHYDROGENASE DEFICIENCY

A 2-year-old child was admitted to a hospital tachypnoeic and looking severely ill. Laboratory tests demonstrated lactic acidosis. After recovery, a detailed examination disclosed a degree of psychomotor retardation. Fibroblasts were taken for culture and the very rare deficiency of PDH was diagnosed. Importantly, in this disorder high-fat, low-carbohydrate diet may improve symptoms.

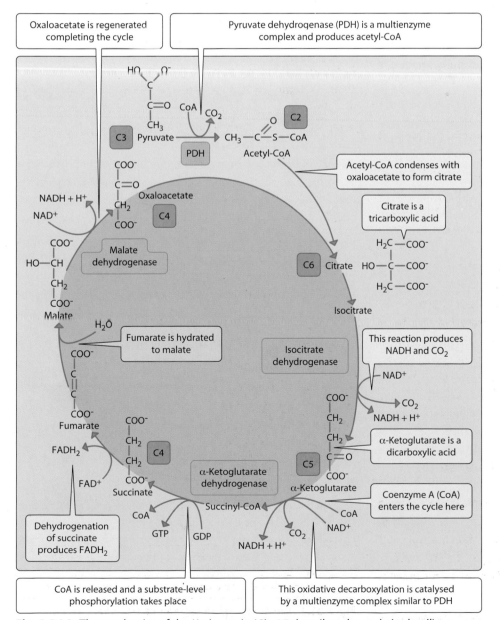

Fig. 3.26.2 The mechanics of the Krebs cycle (Ch. 27 describes the cycle in detail).

27. Krebs cycle (tricarboxylic acid cycle) II

Questions
- What are the control points of the Krebs cycle?
- How does the cycle act as a metabolic hub?

Reactions of the Krebs cycle

The reactions of the Krebs cycle shown in Fig. 3.26.2.

1. The 4-carbon (C4) oxaloacetate condenses with C2 acetyl-CoA to form C6 citrate. This is catalysed by citrate synthase and involves the hydrolysis of the thioester bond.
2. Citrate undergoes dehydration to form aconitate.
3. Aconitate is hydrated by aconitase to form isocitrate.
4. The C6 isocitrate is decarboxylated to C5 α-ketoglutarate by isocitrate dehydrogenase. The reaction yields both NADH and CO_2.
5. The C5 α-ketoglutarate undergoes oxidative decarboxylation to C4 succinyl-CoA by α-ketoglutarate dehydrogenase. NADH and CO_2 are formed. This reaction is catalysed by a multienzyme complex analogous to PDH. From now on, all the metabolites are C4 molecules.
6. Succinyl-CoA is converted to succinate by succinyl-CoA synthetase. This is a substrate-level phosphorylation yielding GTP (which can be converted into ATP).
7. Succinate is oxidized to fumarate by succinate dehydrogenase, an enzyme that sits in the inner mitochondrial membrane; $FADH_2$ is produced and the transported electrons feed into the quinone pool in the respiratory chain.
8. Fumarate is hydrated to malate by fumarase.
9. Malate is oxidized to oxaloacetate by malate dehydrogenase, yielding yet another NADH molecule. This completes the cycle.

Note that the 'cycling' metabolite here is **oxaloacetate**. It condenses with acetyl-CoA at the beginning of the cycle and is regenerated at the completion of a cycle turn. Altogether the cycle produces three hydride ions (6 electrons) that are transferred to NAD^+, and a pair of hydrogen atoms (containing 4 electrons) transferred to FAD.

The overall reaction

The summary reaction of the cycle is:

$$\text{acetyl-CoA} + 3NAD^+ + FAD + GDP + Pi + 2H_2O \rightleftharpoons$$
$$2CO_2 + 3NADH + FADH_2 + GTP + 2H^+ + CoA$$

Energy yield of aerobic glucose metabolism

Aerobic glycolysis

The production of pyruvate from glucose generates 2 ATP per molecule of glucose. When glycolysis proceeds in the presence of O_2, pyruvate is oxidized to acetyl-CoA by PDH, producing 1 molecule of NADH. Another molecule of NADH is produced in the reaction of glyceraldehyde-3-phosphate dehydrogenase. In aerobic conditions, the NADH enters mitochondria, yielding an additional 2.5 molecules of ATP. (Note that 1 molecule of glucose produces 2 molecules of pyruvate via the interconversion of triose phosphates.) The overall energy production per molecule of glucose is:

glycolysis to pyruvate: 2 ATP
2 NADH from glycolysis: 5 ATP
2 NADH from PDH reaction: 5 ATP
oxidation of 2 acetyl-CoA: 20 ATP

Therefore, the total yield of aerobic glycolysis is 32 ATP per molecule of glucose.

Energy yield of the Krebs cycle

NADH is produced in reactions catalysed by PDH, isocitrate dehydrogenase, ketoglutarate dehydrogenase and malate dehydrogenase; $FADH_2$ is produced by succinate dehydrogenase. One molecule of GTP is produced by succinyl-CoA synthetase in a substrate level phosphorylation. So one turn of the cycle produces three molecules of NADH, one of $FADH_2$ and one molecule of GTP (which can be converted to ATP). Assuming the yield of 2.5 molecules of ATP per one NADH oxidized in the respiratory chain and 1.5 ATP per one FADH, the energy yield is:

$$(3 \times 2.5) + 1.5 + 1 = 10$$

Therefore, 10 molecules of ATP are produced by one turn of the cycle. Note that different biochemistry texts calculate this using different yields of ATP from nucleotide oxidation and the values may differ slightly (see Ch. 28).

Regulation

The Krebs cycle

The regulatory enzymes of the cycle are **citrate synthase** and **isocitrate dehydrogenase**. The cycle is inhibited by the high $NADH/NAD^+$ and ATP/ADP ratios. ADP and calcium ion activate isocitrate dehydrogenase. Citrate synthase is controlled by the availability of substrates, oxaloacetate and acetyl-CoA (Fig. 3.27.1).

Regulation of other pathways by Krebs cycle metabolites

Krebs cycle metabolites regulate the rate of glycolysis and fat synthesis. Citrate inhibits phosphofructokinase-1, a key glycolytic enzyme, and stimulates fatty acid synthesis at the malonyl-CoA synthetase level (see p. 37).

The cycle as a metabolic hub

The amphibolic nature of the cycle

The Krebs cycle fulfils amphibolic (both catabolic and anabolic) function. The oxidation of acetyl-CoA is catabolic. The anabolic functions are the contribution to the synthesis of glucose (gluconeogenesis), the provision of acetyl-CoA for fatty acid synthesis and supplying substrates for the synthesis of amino acids, porphyrins and cholesterol.

The anaplerotic reactions

To operate, the cycle needs key metabolites, particularly oxaloacetate. Reactions that replenish metabolites that are constantly consumed are known as anaplerotic (replenishing): for instance, gluconeogenesis is sustained by the degradation of amino acids.

Links with the metabolism of amino acids

Krebs cycle metabolites α-ketoglutarate and oxaloacetate can be transformed into amino acids by transaminations.

Transport of acetyl-CoA out of the mitochondria for use in biosynthetic pathways

When high-energy compounds are abundant in the cell, acetyl-CoA is channelled into the synthesis of fatty acids; however, this takes place in the cytoplasm rather than in mitochondria.

Both ATP and NADH (markers of cellular high-energy status) inhibit the Krebs cycle enzyme **isocitrate dehydrogenase**. This leads to a build-up of citrate and isocitrate. Citrate is transported out of the mitochondria by the **tricarboxylate carrier**. In the cytoplasm, citrate and ATP inhibit glycolysis by inhibiting phosphofructokinase-1 (PFK-1); citrate also stimulates acetyl-CoA carboxylase, the rate-limiting enzyme of lipogenesis. The inhibition of PFK-1 directs glucose into the PPP pathway; this provides NADPH for the biosynthesis of fatty acids. Citrate is cleaved in the cytoplasm by citrate lyase, yielding oxaloacetate and acetyl-CoA, and the acetyl-CoA enters lipogenesis. (See also Ch. 38.)

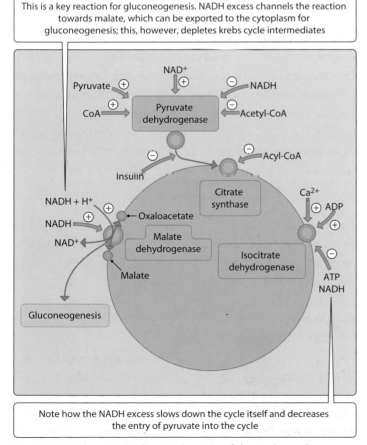

This is a key reaction for gluconeogenesis. NADH excess channels the reaction towards malate, which can be exported to the cytoplasm for gluconeogenesis; this, however, depletes krebs cycle intermediates

Note how the NADH excess slows down the cycle itself and decreases the entry of pyruvate into the cycle

Fig. 3.27.1 The principal control points of the Krebs cycle.

28. The respiratory chain

Questions
- How does copper participate in the electron transfer in complex IV?
- Describe and explain the pH differences between the interior of the mitochondria and the intermembrane space
- What is meant by saying that ATP synthase is a molecular motor?

The respiratory chain provides the infrastructure for movement of electrons from reduced nucleotides to O_2. Reduced nucleotides are derived from cytoplasmic oxidations, transferred into the mitochondrial matrix by metabolic shuttles, and the Krebs cycle, the enzymes of which lie in close proximity to the respiratory chain. The transfer of electrons along the respiratory chain is linked with pumping of hydrogen ions (protons) out from the mitochondrial matrix, creating the proton-motive force. The protons return through the proton channel of **ATP synthase**, driving the synthesis of large amounts of ATP. The combination of oxidative processes with ATP production is **oxidative phosphorylation**. Most of cellular ATP is produced in the respiratory chain. This energy can then be used piecemeal for biosynthetic reactions, thermogenesis, membrane ion transport and production of mechanical energy through muscle contraction.

Location of the respiratory chain

The permeability characteristics of the mitochondrial membranes are highly relevant to the operation of the chain: while the outer membrane is freely permeable to many small molecules and water (it contains a porin), the inner membrane is not, and transporters are required to transfer the molecules from the matrix side to the cytosolic side of the inner mitochondrial membrane. The enzymes of the electron transport chain are embedded in the inner mitochondrial membrane (Fig. 3.28.1). The membrane itself serves as a propagation medium for one of the electron transfer molecules: hydrophobic **coenzyme Q** (CoQ; **ubiquinone**).

The electron-carrying species of the chain are flavins, iron–sulphur clusters (non-haem iron proteins with iron atoms linked to proteins by cysteine residues), quinones, copper ions and haems. The summary reaction of biological oxidations is:

$$2H + \tfrac{1}{2}O_2 \rightleftharpoons H_2O$$

or, taking on account the primary source of electrons in the chain

$$NADH + H^+ + \tfrac{1}{2}O_2 \rightarrow NAD^+ + H_2O$$

The four enzymatic complexes
The redox components of the four large protein complexes are:

- FMN or FAD: complexes I and II
- iron–sulphur clusters: complexes I, II, III
- haems: complexes II, III, IV.

The electron carriers are:

- CoQ: from complexes I and II to complex III
- cytochrome *c*: from complex III to complex IV.

Complex I is NADH-Q reductase. It catalyses the transfer of electrons from NADH to FMN, several iron–sulphur clusters and CoQ. The transfer of four protons from the matrix to the intermembrane space accompanies the reaction:

$$NADH + H^+ + Q \rightleftharpoons NAD^+ + QH_2$$

Next, CoQ diffuses within the membrane to complex III.
Complex II is succinate-Q reductase. This contains succinate dehydrogenase, a Krebs cycle enzyme that is an integral part of the plasma membrane. The complex uses FAD as a prosthetic group; like complex I, it transfers electrons to CoQ but it does not pump protons. CoQ diffuses within the membrane to complex III.
Complex III is Q-cytochrome c oxidoreductase. This enzyme uses CoQ as reductant and transfers electrons to the haem ring of cytochrome *c*. Complex III also contains iron–sulphur

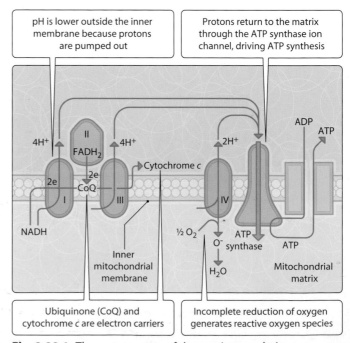

Fig. 3.28.1 The components of the respiratory chain.

clusters and binding sites for CoQ. Complex III pumps two protons from the matrix side. Cytochrome *c* shuttles back and forth to complex IV in the intermembrane space.

Complex IV is cytochrome oxidase. Cytochrome *c* donates electrons to the copper centre within cytochrome oxidase, reducing Cu^{2+} to Cu^+. Electrons are then transferred to several haems and finally to O_2. Complex IV also pumps two protons from the matrix side into the intermembrane space.

Oxidative phosphorylation

The build-up of a proton gradient across the inner mitochondrial membrane stores energy: the outer side of the mitochondrial membrane is 140 mV more positive than the inner side and the pH of the intermembrane space is 1.4 pH units lower than that of the interior. Electron transport is coupled to ATP formation, with protons returning to the matrix via ATP synthase. A flow of three protons is required to synthesize each ATP molecule. As one proton is consumed to transport the ATP out of the mitochondrion, four protons are needed to generate one ATP molecule that is available in the cytoplasm.

The theoretical ATP yield of mitochondrial oxidation is:

- oxidation of 1NADH yields 3ATP
- oxidation of 1FADH$_2$ yields 2ATP.

Taking the energy expenditure associated with transport of ATP to the cytoplasm into account reduces this to:

- 1NADH yields 2.5ATP in the cytoplasm
- 1FADH$_2$ yields 1.5ATP in the cytoplasm.

ATP synthesis

Synthesis of ATP is catalysed by the mitochondrial ATPase (ATP synthase) (Fig. 3.28.2). This enzyme complex has catalytic subunits (F_1) located on the inner side of the inner mitochondrial membrane and a proton channel (F_0) that spans the membrane. ATP synthase is a molecular motor; the transport of protons through the channel drives the rotation of its subunits and the formation of ATP from ADP. Formed ATP is exported to the cytoplasm via membrane transport in exchange for ADP.

Inhibitors and uncouplers

The activity of the respiratory chain can be inhibited at different levels (Fig. 3.28.3). Mitochondrial oxidation reactions can be uncoupled from phosphorylation by **uncoupling protein-1 (thermogenin)**. The produced energy is then released as heat. In brown fat, this is important for thermogenesis (e.g. in hibernating animals). Thermogenin is also stimulated by thyroxine.

Regulation of the respiratory chain

The rate of oxidative phosphorylation is mainly determined by the supply of ADP (the ATP/ADP ratio also determines the activity of the Krebs cycle and of glycolysis). Thus the activity of the energy-producing pathways depends on the cellular energy charge. In the 'energized' cell, energy production slows down, whereas in the energy-starved cell the main fuel pathways operate at a greater rate. Defects in the electron transport chain are very rare but can lead to myopathy, encephalopathy (Leigh disease) and developmental retardation.

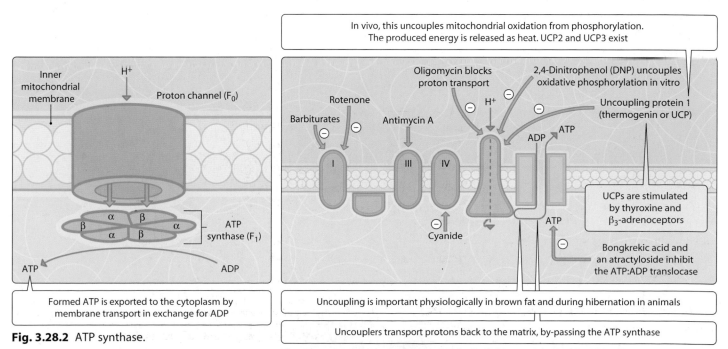

Fig. 3.28.2 ATP synthase.

Fig. 3.28.3 Inhibitors and uncouplers of the respiratory chain.

29. Metabolic shuttles

Questions
- What is the biological significance of metabolic shuttles?
- Which of the shuttles involves transamination reactions?
- Can citrate cross the mitochondrial membrane?

The cell is divided into compartments separated by the lipid bilayer plasma membrane. The membranes are permeable to water because of pores (aquaporins) that allow water passage. However, the inner mitochondrial membrane is only selectively permeable to small molecules yet cellular metabolism necessitates transport of compounds between cellular compartments. The compounds that need to be transported are the reduced nucleotides NADH and NADPH, produced in the cytoplasm, which need to reach the respiratory chain, and also acetyl-CoA,

generated in the mitochondria but serves as a substrate for biosynthetic reactions in the cytoplasm.

Transport of reducing equivalents to the mitochondria
Two metabolic shuttles transport reducing equivalents to the mitochondria, bypassing the need for a specific NADH transport system.

The glycerol phosphate shuttle. This shuttle (Fig. 3.29.1) helps to carry electrons from the cytoplasm into the mitochondrion in muscle. It constitutes a sequence of reactions where the initial step is the reduction of dihydroxyacetone phosphate (DHAP), a glycolytic metabolite, by NADH, yielding glycerol 3-phosphate. Glycerol 3-phosphate is oxidized at

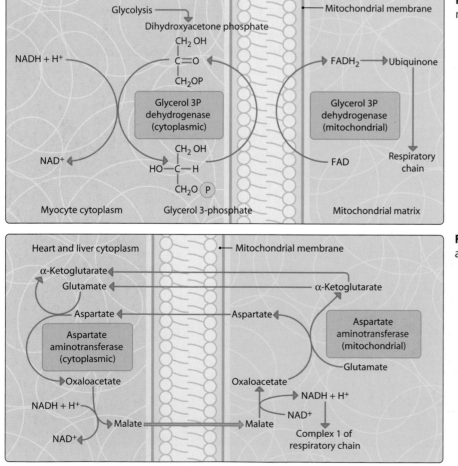

Fig. 3.29.1 The glycerol phosphate shuttle in muscle.

Fig. 3.29.2 The malate–asparate shuttle in heart and liver.

the inner mitochondrial membrane by the mitochondrial glycerol-3-phosphate dehydrogenase, which yields $FADH_2$; the $FADH_2$ can then donate electrons to coenzyme Q in the respiratory chain.

The malate–aspartate shuttle. This shuttle (Fig. 3.29.2) operates in the liver and in heart muscle. Oxaloacetate cannot cross the inner mitochondrial membrane and so it is reduced in the cytoplasm to malate. Malate is transported across the membrane and is reconverted to oxaloacetate, yielding NADH. The mitochondrial oxaloacetate undergoes transamination with glutamate, generating aspartate and α-ketoglutarate. Aspartate is transported out of the mitochondria and is either deaminated or transaminated to yield oxaloacetate, closing the cycle. This shuttle operates when the concentration of NADH is higher in the cytosol than in the mitochondria.

Transport of acetyl-CoA to the cytoplasm

The pyruvate–malate shuttle supplies acetyl-CoA for biosynthetic reactions in the cytoplasm (Fig. 3.29.3). This shuttle allows the transport of acetyl-CoA out of the mitochondria. Acetyl-CoA is converted to citrate, which is transported across the inner mitochondrial membrane by the tricarboxylate carrier. In the cytoplasm, citrate is cleaved into acetyl-CoA and oxaloacetate by citrate lyase. Oxaloacetate is reduced to malate, and malate undergoes oxidative decarboxylation by the malic enzyme, yielding pyruvate and CO_2. Pyruvate can re-enter the mitochondrial matrix. Incidentally, the malic enzyme reaction provides as much as 40% of cytoplasmic NADPH for fatty acid synthesis. The other 60% comes from the pentose phosphate pathway (see Ch. 30).

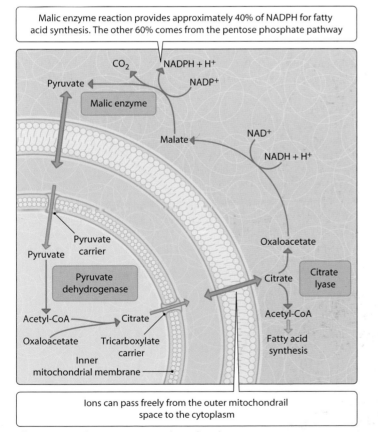

Fig. 3.29.3 The pyruvate–malate shuttle.

30. The pentose phosphate pathway and metabolism of sugars other than glucose

Questions
- Which electron carrier molecule is involved in the reactions of the pentose phosphate pathway?
- What are the types of reaction involved in the transfer of 2- and 3-carbon units between molecules?
- At which stage do the metabolites of fructose enter glycolysis?

The cytosolic pentose phosphate pathway (PPP) branches off from glycolysis (in fact, it shortcuts part of it) (Fig. 3.30.1). It is an oxidative pathway active in the liver, erythrocytes, adipose tissue, adrenal cortex, testis, thyroid and mammary gland. Its importance is that it produces NADPH (not NADH), which is needed for biosynthetic reactions in the cytoplasm such as the synthesis of fatty acids and steroids (including cholesterol), and also for the reduction of glutathione. It also produces ribose 5-phosphate, a sugar essential for the synthesis of nucleotides and nucleic acids.

The PPP is stimulated when glucose is plentiful (e.g. with carbohydrate-rich diet). In such conditions, there is plenty of pyruvate to supply the Krebs cycle, and the accumulating citrate inhibits phosphofructokinase-1 (PFK-1); this redirects glucose 6-phosphate (Glc6P) into the PPP.

The pentose phosphate pathway

The first step is the oxidation of Glc6P by Glc6P dehydrogenase (Glc6PDH; a NADP$^+$-dependent enzyme) to 6-phosphoglucono-D-lactone, then by 6-phosphogluconate dehydrogenase (also NADP$^+$ dependent) and decarboxylated by 6-phosphogluconate dehydrogenase to the 5-carbon ribulose 5-phosphate. This stage produces two molecules of NADPH.

Ribulose 5-phosphate is then transformed into ribose 5-phosphate and xylulose 5-phosphate. Several other transfers of 2-carbon and 3-carbon units (see below) take place, finally yielding fructose 6-phosphate (F6P), and glyceraldehyde 3-phosphate. Both compounds rejoin glycolysis. Fructose 1-phosphate (F1P) and ribulose 5-phosphate can be converted to Glc6P (Fig. 3.24.1).

Metabolism of 2- and 3-carbon intermediates

Transketolase transfers 2-carbon units from a ketose onto the aldehyde carbon of an aldose. It uses magnesium and thiamine as cofactors:

ribose-5P (C5) + xylulose-5P (C5) $\rightleftharpoons$ sedoheptulose-7P (C7)
and glyceraldehyde-3P (C3)

Transaldolase transfers 3-carbon units from sedoheptulose 7-phosphate to glyceraldehyde 3-phosphate to form F6P and erythrose 4-phosphate. Thus:

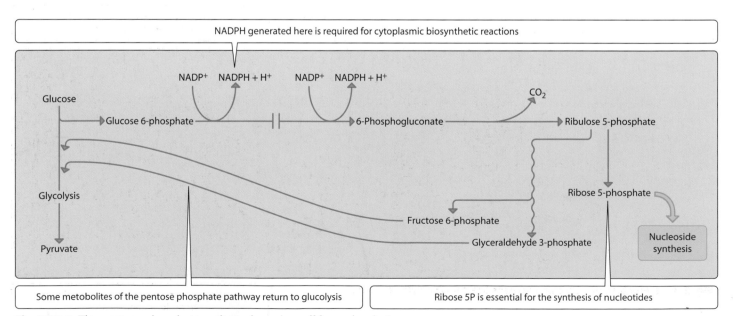

NADPH generated here is required for cytoplasmic biosynthetic reactions

Some metabolites of the pentose phosphate pathway return to glycolysis

Ribose 5P is essential for the synthesis of nucleotides

Fig. 3.30.1 The pentose phosphate pathway branches off from glycolysis.

sedoheptulose-7P (C7) + glyceraldehyde-3P (C3) $\rightleftharpoons$

$$F6P + \text{erythrose-4P (C4)}$$

These reactions may proceed in either direction.

Regulation of the pentose phosphate pathway

The PPP is regulated by NADPH, which inhibits its regulatory enzyme, Glc6PDH.

Metabolic conversions of sugars other than glucose

Glucose, fructose and galactose are the main hexoses absorbed in the gastrointestinal tract. Fructose and galactose are released from sucrose and lactose, respectively, and both can be transformed to glucose. These considerations are important for nutrition and in calculating caloric intake. Note that glucose is not the only easily metabolizable simple monosaccharide in the diet.

Fructose

Fructose is converted to F1P by fructokinase. Next, F1P is cleaved to glyceraldehyde and dihydroxyacetone phosphate (DHAP) by aldolase B (an enzyme that also cleaves fructose 1,6-bisphosphate) (Fig. 3.30.2). D-Glyceraldehyde is phosphorylated by thiokinase to glyceraldehyde 3-phosphate. The two triose phosphates, DHAP and glyceraldehyde 3-phosphate, enter glycolysis (or gluconeogenesis). Note that the pathway of fructose metabolism bypasses the regulatory step of PFK-1. Thus the ingestion of excess fructose may lead to increased fatty acid and triacylglycerol synthesis (and to weight gain).

Amino sugars can be synthesized from F6P. The first reaction is transamination with glutamine, yielding D-glucosamine 6-phosphate. Acetylations and formation of a UDP-derivative follow. This pathway leads to the synthesis of glucosamine, galactosamine, mannosamine and sialic acid and is important in the synthesis of glycoproteins, glycosphingolipids and glycosaminoglycans (see Ch. 19).

Galactose

Galactokinase phosphorylates galactose to galactose 1-phosphate (Fig. 3.30.3). Galactose 1-phosphate can be converted to glucose 1-phosphate by galactose-1-phosphate uridyltransferase, with the participation of UDP:

$$\text{Gal-1P} + \text{UDPGlc} \rightleftharpoons \text{UDPGal and G1P}$$

UDP-galactose-4-epimerase can then liberate glucose. Galactose may also be formed from glucose. In the lactating mammary gland, UDP-galactose condenses with glucose to yield lactose (this is catalysed by lactose synthase). Galactose is a component of cerebrosides proteoglycans and glycoproteins.

 HEREDITARY FRUCTOSE INTOLERANCE

A 6-month-old baby became drowsy after bottle-feeding and laboratory testing demonstrated hypoglycaemia and lactic acidosis; there was non-glucose reducing substances but no glucose in urine. Hereditary fructose intolerance—deficiency of fructose 1-phosphate aldolase—was diagnosed. In this disorder, fructose cannot be converted to glucose, hence the hypoglycaemia.

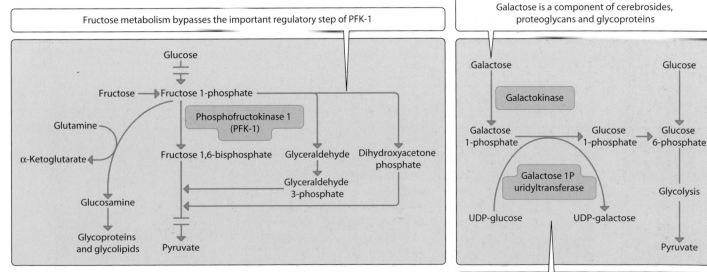

Fig. 3.30.2 Fructose metabolism bypasses the key glycolytic reaction.

Fig. 3.30.3 Galactose is converted to a glycolytic intermediate.

31. Glycogen I: metabolism

Questions
- Why is glycogen an important energy store?
- What is the basic structure of glycogen?
- How is glucose activated to allow its polymerization?

Brain, in normal circumstances, uses glucose as its only fuel. It is, therefore, essential that appropriate levels of glucose are always present in blood (normal glucose concentration is between 3.5 and 5 mmol/l, and symptomatic hypoglycaemia is likely to develop when glucose concentration falls below 2.5 mmol/l). Further, the 'fight and flight' reaction requires an instant supply of metabolic fuel for muscle. Glycogen provides such short-term emergency fuel supply and so is a vital part of the organism's survival system.

Glycogen is a branched polymer of α-D-glucose and is present both in the liver and in muscle. It is normally replenished during feeding under the influence of insulin. Liver glycogen is an emergency store that sustains the blood glucose concentration. Muscle glycogen provides local fuel only as it lacks glucose-6-phosphatase. Not surprisingly, regulatory mechanisms differ between these two tissues.

The key points of glycogen synthesis are:

- a protein glycogenin in each glycogen molecule acts as a primer to initiate its synthesis; it catalyses the addition of the first few glucose molecules to a tyrosine residue in the protein
- the glucose units come directly from UDP-glucose
- glucose molecules are added at the non-reducing end of the primer to give α-1–4 links
- a branching enzyme adds the 1–6 linkages.

The key points of glycogen breakdown are:

- glycogen phosphorylase acts at the multiple non-reducing ends to form glucose 1-phosphate
- many branches means there are many such ends and glucose 1-phosphate is produced rapidly
- debranching enzyme allows complete utilization of glycogen.

Synthesis of glycogen (glycogenogenesis)
Glucose is phosphorylated in the cell by hexokinase (or, in the liver, by its isoform glucokinase) (Fig. 3.31.1). Next, phosphoglucomutase transforms glucose 6-phosphate into glucose 1-phosphate,

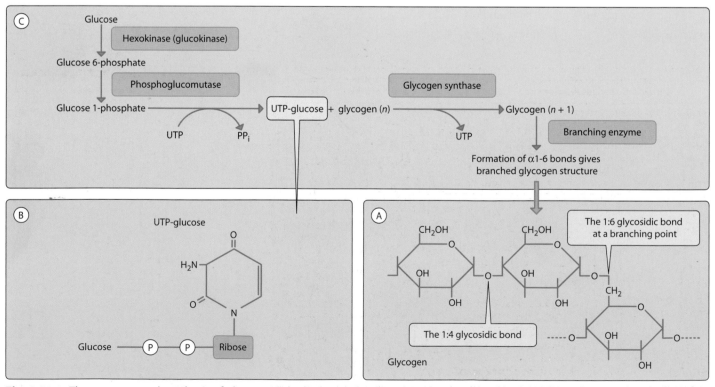

Fig. 3.31.1 The structure and synthesis of glycogen.

which reacts with UTP to give UDP-glucose and pyrophosphate (catalysed by UDP-glucose pyrophosphorylase).

Glycogen synthase joins the C1 of UDP-glucose with the C4 of the terminal residue of existing glycogen (forming a 1–4 glycosidic bond), releasing UDP. A primer, glycogenin, is necessary to initiate glycogen synthesis. The glycogen chain is constructed in a linear fashion until it reaches 11 glucose residues in length; at that point, **branching enzyme** transfers several 1,4–linked units to form a branch linked through the 1–6 bond.

Degradation of glycogen (glycogenolysis)

The structure of glycogen, with many end-residues exposed on the surface, enables access by many enzyme molecules at the same time.

Degradation of glycogen is catalysed by **glycogen phosphorylase**, which yields glucose 1-phosphate (Fig. 3.31.2), which is then converted to glucose 6-phosphate. The release of glucose into the circulation requires the presence of glucose-6-phosphatase. Liver and kidney (but not muscle) possess this enzyme.

The 1–6 branches of glycogen are degraded by a **debranching enzyme**. Hydrolysis of 1–6 bond is carried out by a 1,6-glucosidase (part of the bifunctional debranching enzyme).

Glycogen stores become depleted after a 12–18 h fast (see Ch. 51).

Fig. 3.31.2 Release of glucose from glycogen.

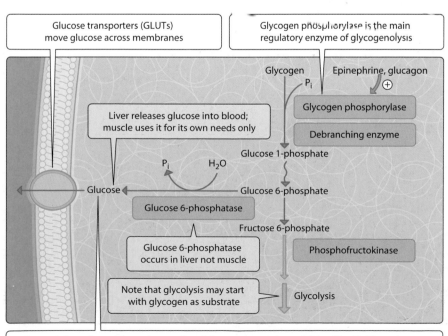

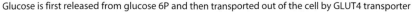

32. Glycogen II: regulation of metabolism

Questions
- How does glycogen synthesis and degradation reflect the balance between anabolic and catabolic hormones?
- How are glycogen synthase and glycogen phosphorylase affected by phosphorylation?
- What is the role of cAMP in glycogen degradation?

Mechanisms of regulation

It is essential to consider the control of the synthetic and degradation pathways for glycogen together. The two controlling enzymes, glycogen synthase and glycogen phosphorylase, are regulated by phosphorylation/dephosphorylation reactions driven by hormonal signals (Fig. 3.32.1). These are opposing systems:

- glycogen phosphorylase (glycogen breakdown) is activated by phosphorylation
- glycogen synthase (glycogen synthesis) is activated by dephosphorylation.

In muscle, cAMP-dependent protein kinase A phosphorylates **phosphorylase kinase**, activating it. Calcium ions also activate this enzyme. Activated phosphorylase kinase phosphorylates glycogen phosphorylase: this phosphorylation transforms the enzyme from its inactive (phosphorylase b) to its active (phosphorylase a) form. This thiamin-dependent enzyme is the key step in glycogenolysis. It is dephosphorylated by protein phosphatase-1, which returns it to the b form.

In contrast to glycogen phosphorylase, glycogen synthase is active when dephosphorylated. It is phosphorylated (and thus inhibited) by both cAMP-dependent and calcium-dependent kinases.

Dephosphorylation is accomplished by the protein phosphatase-1, controlled by cAMP-dependent protein kinase A. This phosphatase also controls dephosphorylation of phosphorylase a, phosphorylase kinase a and glycogen synthase; the overall effect is activating glycogen synthesis and inhibiting glycogenolysis.

Hormonal control

Insulin, on the one hand, and glucagon and epinephrine, on the other, are the principal regulators of glycogen synthesis and degradation:

- glucagon: stimulation of glycogenolysis in liver
- epinephrine: stimulation of glycogenolysis in muscle
- cortisol: weaker stimulation of glycogenolysis
- insulin: inhibition of glycogenolysis.

Decreasing glucose concentration, as well as the 'fight and flight' reaction, stimulates secretion of epinephrine and glucagon and suppresses insulin. Epinephrine and glucagon act instantly to replenish blood glucose from glycogen stores. The glucagon receptor is coupled to G-proteins and to adenylyl cyclase (Fig. 3.32.1). Production of cAMP activates protein kinase A, which initiates further phosphorylations. Epinephrine acts on α_1-adrenoceptors and activates phosphorylase kinase through cAMP-independent mobilization of calcium ions. Insulin inhibits activation of phosphorylase by increasing the concentration of an inhibitor of the enzyme, glucose 6-phosphate.

In addition, the concentrations of several metabolites affect glycogen metabolism. For instance, glycogen synthesis is stimulated by glucose in the liver. In muscle, glycogen breakdown is stimulated by AMP and suppressed by ATP; glucose 6-phosphate inhibits glycogenolysis and stimulates glycogen synthesis in muscle.

Muscle lacks glucose 6-phosphatase and so the end-product of glycogen in muscle is pyruvate (and lactate) from glycolysis. In liver, which does contain glucose 6-phosphatase, the end product is glucose, which can be released into the bloodstream. The localization of an enzyme allows the two tissues to utilize glycogen in distinct ways: muscle using it as an energy source to provide its ATP and liver using it to maintain blood glucose levels. This is known as the glucose–lactate cycle (Fig. 3.32.2).

GLYCOGEN STORAGE DISEASES

Glycogen storage diseases are inborn deficiencies of enzymes of glycogen metabolism. They result in the accumulation of abnormal type or quantity of glycogen, or difficulties with glycogen release. They include deficiencies of glucose-6-phosphatase (type I, von Gierke's disease), muscle phosphorylase (type V, McArdle's disease) and also branching (type IV) and debranching enzyme (type III).

Glycogen storage disease type I
A 5-month-old baby suffered a seizure and developed hypoglycaemia between feeding times. She had a protuberant abdomen, truncal obesity and a moderate hepatomegaly and liver biopsy demonstrated a large degree of glycogen accumulation. She had glycogen storage disease type I.

Glycogen storage disease type V
A 17-year-old boy could tolerate only mild exercise. After attempting to play football, he passed a wine-coloured urine and was sent to the hospital. His blood creatine kinase (see p. 000) was 12 000 U/l (normal < 210 U/l) and he had myoglobinuria. He was diagnosed as having glycogen storage disease type V. His acute episode was caused by the destruction of muscle cells (rhabdomyolysis). The danger of rhabdomyolysis is that it can cause renal failure.

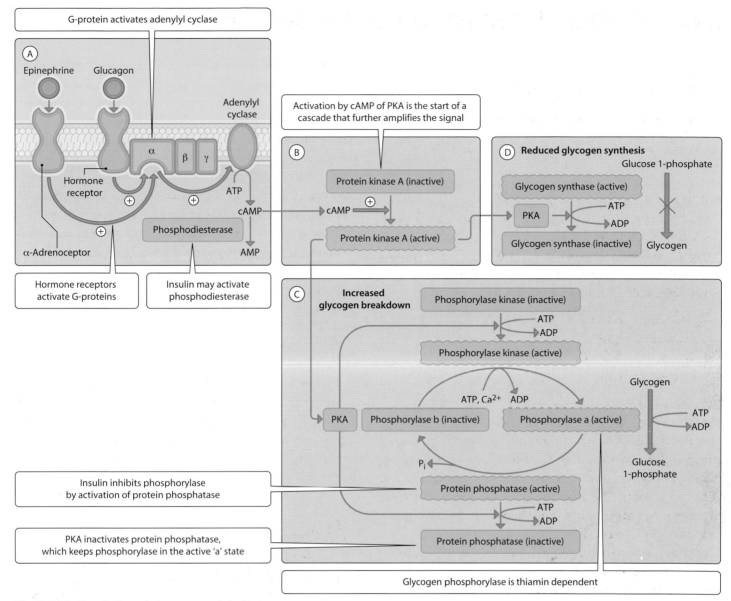

Fig. 3.32.1 Regulation of glycogen metabolism.

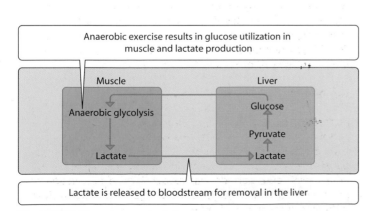

Fig. 3.32.2 The glucose–lactate cycle.

33. Gluconeogenesis I: the pathway

Questions
- In what ways is gluconeogenesis not simply a reversal of glycolysis?
- What are the main gluconeogenic substrates?

Gluconeogenesis is the pathway of glucose synthesis from non-carbohydrate sources. Although glucose is constantly needed to support brain function, liver glycogen stores last for only a few hours—and can be depleted even after a fast as short as overnight. This is where gluconeogenesis comes in (Fig. 3.33.1).

Substrates for gluconeogenesis

The three most important substrates for gluconeogenesis are the amino acid **alanine**, the glycolytic metabolite **lactate** and a lipid, **glycerol** (Fig. 3.33.1).

Alanine in this context serves also as a means for the conversion of other amino acids to glucose (other amino acids can be converted into alanine by transamination). Therefore, when an organism becomes glucose depleted, muscle proteins are used as fuel. It can be regarded as using up a reserve; however, if gluconeogenesis progresses for a long time damage to structural proteins ensues. Consequently, excessive gluconeogenesis over a long period of time is not desirable. The **glucose-alanine cycle** describes movement of alanine produced in muscle to the liver. In the fasting state, gluconeogenesis from alanine will allow increased glucose secretion into the bloodstream for use as a fuel in the brain and in muscle. The process also occurs in exercise.

Glycerol

It is helpful to link gluconeogenesis with the oxidation of fatty acids. Note that lipolysis provides one of the gluconeogenic

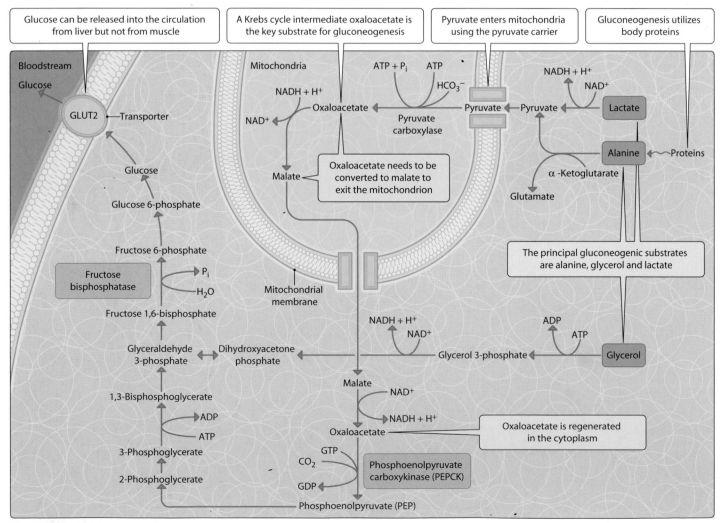

Fig. 3.33.1 Gluconeogenesis.

substrates, glycerol. Also, beta-oxidation of fatty acids is a source of large amounts of acetyl-CoA and NADPH, and therefore ATP. This ATP is made available for use in the key reactions of gluconeogenesis catalysed by **pyruvate carboxylase**, **phosphoenolpyruvate carboxykinase** (PEPCK) and **phosphoglycerate kinase**.

Lactate

During vigerous exercise, muscle becomes anaerobic and the end-product of glycolysis is lactate. The lactate is released into the bloodstream and converted to glucose by the liver. This glucose can then return to muscle for fuel.

Sequence of reactions

Although gluconeogenesis produces glucose, it is not just a reversal of glycolysis (Fig. 3.33.1). The three key reactions of glycolysis that proceed with a large negative free energy change are bypassed during gluconeogenesis by using different enzymes. These three are

- pyruvate kinase: bypassed by PEPCK
- phosphofructokinase-1 (PFK-1): bypassed by fructose 1,6-bisphosphatase (fructose 1,6-bisphosphatase)
- hexokinase/glucokinase: bypassed by glucose-6-phosphatase.

In addition, the key gluconeogenetic intermediate, **oxaloacetate**, must be transported out of the mitochondria. This is accomplished by the malate–oxaloacetate shuttle (Ch. 29). Oxaloacetate is reduced to malate, which is transported out of the mitochondria by the dicarboxylate carrier. Next, malate is reoxidized to oxaloacetate. Now oxaloacetate undergoes GTP-dependent decarboxylation by PEPCK to yield phosphoenolpyruvate (PEP). High glucagon concentration and alanine inhibit pyruvate kinase, directing PEP into gluconeogenesis rather than glycolysis.

From the PEP stage on, the pathway runs as a reversal of glycolysis through enolase, 2-phosphoglycerate mutase, phosphoglycerate kinase (ATP-requiring), glyceraldehyde-3-phosphate dehydrogenase (NADH) and aldolase, yielding fructose 1,6-bisphosphate. Note that the aldolase reaction uses dihydroacetone phosphate, a metabolite of glycerol (this is the entry point for glycerol into gluconeogenesis).

34. Gluconeogenesis II: regulation

Questions
- What are the regulatory enzymes of gluconeogenesis?
- What effect does excess alcohol intake have on gluconeogenesis?

Regulatory steps

Because glycolysis and gluconeogenesis have many enzymes in common and are opposing pathways, a precise control mechanism is required to ensure that glucose formation and utilization occurs when and where the body requires. The two pathways are controlled by:

- allosteric effector molecules
- covalent modification of enzymes
- alterations in enzyme concentrations.

There are three control points (Figs 3.34.1 and 3.34.2):

- between phosphoenolpyruvate and pyruvate
- between fructose 1,6-bisphophate and fructose 6-phosphate
- between glucose 6-phosphate and glucose.

Phosphoenolpyruvate to pyruvate

The formation of phosphoenolpyruvate from pyruvate requires two enzymes: pyruvate carboxylase utilizes ATP and has an absolute requirement for acetyl-CoA as an allosteric activator and phosphoenolpyruvate carboxykinase uses GTP. In addition oxaloacetate has to be transferred out of the mitochondria (Chs 29 and 33).

Although acetyl-CoA is not itself converted into glucose, it does affect the rate of gluconeogenesis by its regulatory effects. Abundance of acetyl-CoA decreases the activity of isocitrate dehydrogenase; this slows down the Krebs cycle. Acetyl-CoA decreases the activity of pyruvate dehydrogenase, controlling its own formation from pyruvate. Also, the activity of pyruvate carboxylase, and thus the conversion of pyruvate into oxaloacetate, increases. These conditions favour a build-up of oxaloacetate and its channelling away from the Krebs cycle into gluconeogenesis.

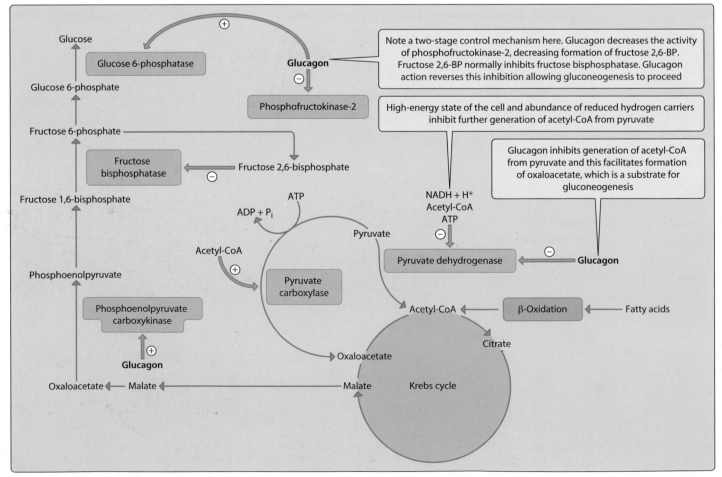

Fig. 3.34.1 Control of gluconeogenesis.

Fructose 1,6-bisphosphate to fructose 6-phosphate

The second important regulatory point of gluconeogenesis is **fructose 1,6-bisphosphatase**. It is controlled by glucagon and fructose 2,6-bisphosphate, a product of the reaction catalysed by phosphofructokinase (PFK)-2, which we are now familiar with (compare with Ch. 24). As fructose 2,6-bisphosphate inhibits fructose 1,6-bisphosphatase, it will inhibit gluconeogenesis. Glucagon stimulates fructose 2,6-bisphosphatase, the enzyme that hydrolyses fructose 2,6-bisphosphate; the decrease in fructose 2,6-bisphosphate will remove its inhibition of fructose 1,6-bisphosphatase, allowing gluconeogenesis to proceed. Glucagon also inhibits PFK-1 and, therefore, glycolysis.

Glucose 6-phosphate to glucose

Finally in gluconeogenesis, glucose-6-phosphatase present in the endoplasmic reticulum liberates glucose from glucose 6-phosphate. Glucose is transported by the glucose transporter GLUT7 from the endoplasmic reticulum to the cytoplasm, and then by GLUT4 across the cell membrane to the extracellular fluid.

Role of glucagon in regulation of gluconeogenesis

Glucagon coordinates activity of several pathways (Fig. 3.26.2). It is a major stimulator of both gluconeogenesis and lipolysis. Its action promotes gluconeogenesis by a direct effect on the enzymes of the pathway and also by adjustments in the other major pathways. In addition to increasing the activities of pyruvate kinase, PEPCK and glucose-6-phosphatase, glucagon increases the activity of hormone-sensitive lipase in the adipose tissue. Glucagon also increases the synthesis of aminotransferases, providing the supply of alanine for gluconeogenesis.

Relation of gluconeogenesis with other pathways

Lipolysis

Glycerol generated by hydrolysis of triacylglycerols can be phosphorylated in the liver to glycerol 3-phosphate, and then oxidized to dihydroxyacetone phosphate.

The long-held view has been that other products of lipolysis, the fatty acids, cannot be converted into glucose. The argument has been that because acetyl-CoA, a product of beta-oxidation of the fatty acids, enters the Krebs cycle as a 2-carbon unit there is no net synthesis because these two carbons are lost as CO_2 during the cycle. This, however, cannot be entirely accurate as isotopic studies do show traces of acetyl-CoA carbons in newly synthesized glucose.

Ketogenesis

Gluconeogenesis depletes the Krebs cycle of oxaloacetate and so any excess of acetyl-CoA cannot condense with oxaloacetate to form citrate; in such conditions acetyl-CoA enters ketogenesis (Ch. 36).

Protein-sparing action of glucose

Administering glucose to a patient who relies on gluconeogenesis to maintain blood glucose concentration stimulates insulin secretion and increases the insulin-to-glucagon ratio. This inhibits gluconeogenesis and decreases the transamination reactions that supply alanine for gluconeogenesis. The result is sparing muscle proteins from degradation. This is known as the protein-sparing action of glucose.

 EFFECTS OF ALCOHOL

A man in his fifties was admitted to hospital mid-morning strongly smelling of alcohol. He had abnormal liver function tests, a glucose concentration of 2.2 mmol/l (adult reference range 4–6 mmol/l) and diabetes mellitus was excluded. Alcohol inhibits gluconeogenesis; alcohol excess, together with poor food intake, may precipitate hypoglycaemia.

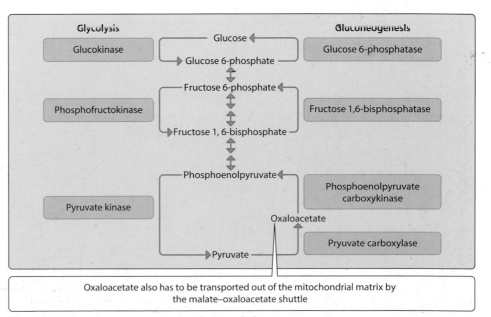

Fig. 3.34.2 Regulatory steps in glycolysis and gluconeogenesis.

35. Lipolysis and beta-oxidation of fatty acids

Questions
- How is hormone-sensitive lipase regulated?
- What is meant by the term 'activation of a fatty acid'?
- How is fatty acyl-CoA transported across the mitochondrial membrane?

Degradation of neutral fat (triacylglycerols) is another key pathway in energy metabolism; it sustains the organism when food is not readily available. It is particularly important in prolonged fasting or exercise.

Lipolysis
Triacylglycerols are hydrolysed to glycerol and fatty acids by hormone-sensitive lipase (Fig. 3.35.1), activated (much like glycogen phosphorylase) by cAMP-dependent phosphorylation and, therefore, responding to glucagon and epinephrine. Insulin inhibits lipolysis. Glycerol is transported to the liver, phosphorylated by **glycerol kinase** and may be further oxidized to dihydroxyacetone phosphate to be converted to a glycolytic metabolite glyceraldehyde 3-phosphate. Fatty acids are transferred to the liver where they are activated by **acyl-CoA synthetase** to yield **acyl-CoA** for further oxidation.

Beta-oxidation of fatty acids
Transport of acyl groups to the mitochondrial matrix: carnitine
Beta-oxidation takes place in the mitochondrial matrix but acyl-

CoAs cannot cross the inner mitochondrial membrane. Fatty acids are transported across the membrane bound to an alcohol, carnitine (Fig. 3.35.2). **Carnitine palmitoyltransferase I** catalyses the formation of acylcarnitine on the outside of membrane; the acylcarnitine moves across the membrane and the acyl residue then is transferred to mitochondrial CoA on the matrix side of the membrane (catalysed by carnitine palmitoyltransferase II). Carnitine returns to repeat the cycle, and acyl-CoA enters mitochondrial oxidation.

Mitochondrial oxidation
In the mitochondrial matrix, acyl-CoA is degraded to 2-carbon fragments in a cyclical sequence of four reactions (Fig. 3.35.3).

1. *Oxidation by FAD.* Acyl-CoA dehydrogenase uses FAD as its electron acceptor.
2. *Hydration.* Catalysed by L-3-hydroxyacyl-CoA dehydrogenase.
3. *Oxidation by NAD+.* The second oxidation by NAD^+ is catalysed by hydroxyacyl-CoA dehydrogenase.
4. *Thiolysis.* This reaction splits the original molecule to give acetyl-CoA (C2) and an acyl-CoA that is shorter by a 2-carbon unit.

The shortened acyl-CoA re-enters the cycle. A further seven cycles would be required to degrade a molecule of the most common fatty acid, palmitate (C16). Because the oxidation affects the β-carbon, the process is known as beta-oxidation.

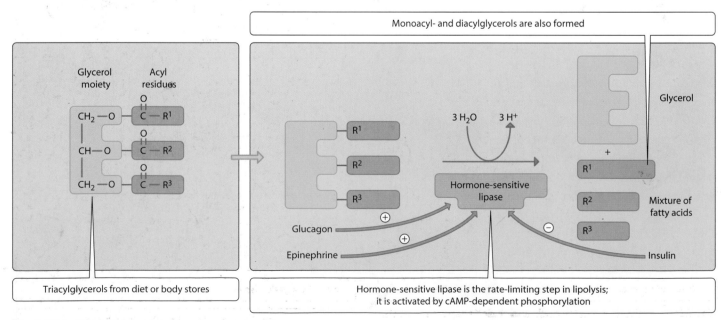

Fig. 3.35.1 Lipolysis.

(Handwritten annotation: "on then enter the Krebs cycle")

This pathway is modified when very long, short, or unsaturated fatty acids, are degraded. Three different acyl-CoA dehydrogenases oxidize the long-chain (C12–C18), medium-chain (C4–C14) and short-chain (C4–C6) fatty acids. Some very-long-chain fatty acids are oxidized in peroxisomes rather than mitochondria: there, the flavoprotein dehydrogenase transfers electrons to O_2 instead of the respiratory chain. This yields H_2O_2, which is converted by catalase to water and molecular O_2. These reactions shorten the very-long-chain fatty acid chains until they are ready for 'conventional' beta-oxidation.

The oxidation of unsaturated fatty acids requires two new enzymes, an isomerase and a 2,4-dienoyl-CoA reductase to reconfigure bonds to permit beta-oxidation. The odd-numbered fatty acids yield acetyl-CoA and propionyl-CoA. Propionyl-CoA is converted to the succinyl-CoA in one of two reactions in the body that require vitamin B_{12} as coenzyme.

The overall reaction in beta-oxidation
Using palmitoyl acid (C16) as an example, the overall reaction of beta-oxidation is:

palmitoyl-CoA + 7FAD + 7NAD⁺ + 7CoA + 7H₂O ⇌
8acetyl-CoA 7FADH₂ + 7NADH + 7H⁺

The energy yield of beta-oxidation
The oxidation of a 16-carbon molecule produces 8 acetyl-CoA, 7 NADH and 7 FADH₂. Assuming the yield of 2.5 molecules of ATP per 1 NADH oxidized in the respiratory chain and 1.5 ATP per 1 FADH, the energy yield is: $(7 \times 2.5) + (7 \times 1.5) = 28ATP$. The 8 molecules of acetyl-CoA oxidized in the Krebs cycle would each yield 10 ATP, giving 80 ATP. Two ATP are used to activate the fatty acid; therefore, the overall yield is 106 ATP molecules.

Beta-oxidation and ketogenesis
Importantly, the entry of acetyl-CoA into the Krebs cycle depends on the availability of oxaloacetate. If oxaloacetate is not available, acetyl-CoA is directed into ketogenesis (compare Chs 27 and 38).

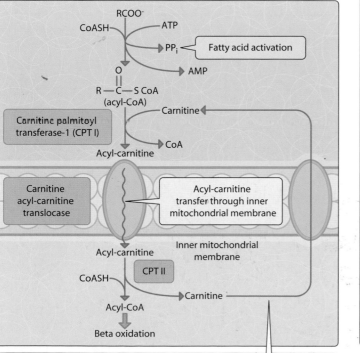

Fig. 3.35.2 Activation of fatty acids and their transport across the inner mitochondrial membrane.

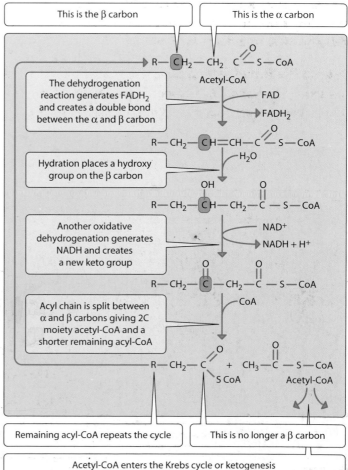

Fig. 3.35.3 Beta-oxidation of fatty acids.

36. Ketogenesis

Questions

- Which organs are involved in ketogenesis?
- Which metabolite is common for ketogenesis and cholesterol synthesis?
- In which clinical conditions is ketonaemia present?

Ketogenesis is a short pathway closely linked to lipolysis and gluconeogenesis. It is important in long-term fasting and in poorly controlled diabetes mellitus. It plays a role in the fuel metabolism as means of recycling CoA.

Ketone bodies derive from acetyl-CoA. They are acetoacetate, β-hydroxybutyrate and acetone (Fig. 3.36.1). Ketogenesis takes place in the liver, but its indirect substrates, fatty acids, are also generated in the adipose tissue by hormone-sensitive lipase.

Ketogenesis and substrate supply

Ketogenesis is activated when there is an excess of acetyl-CoA (Fig. 3.36.2). This happens during fasting, when active gluco-neogenesis depletes the Krebs cycle of oxaloacetate. Because the entry of acetyl-CoA into the cycle does depend on the availability of oxaloacetate, when oxaloacetate becomes sparse an excess of acetyl-CoA builds up and is channelled into ketogenesis in the liver.

Reactions of ketogenesis

Acetyl-CoA thiolase converts acetyl-CoA to acetoacetyl-CoA and subsequently to hydroxymethylglutaryl (HMG)-CoA (this releases two CoA molecules) (Fig. 3.36.3). Next, HMG-CoA is cleaved into acetoacetate and acetyl-CoA by HMG-CoA lyase. Acetoacetate may be reduced by NADH to β-3-hydroxybutyrate or it can be non-enzymatically decarboxylated to acetone.

Ketone bodies and the metabolism of amino acids

The metabolism of some amino acids also produces acetyl-CoA or HMG-CoA: these amino acids are called **ketogenic** (as opposed to **glucogenic**) (Table 3.36.1). Some amino acids can be both glucogenic and ketogenic.

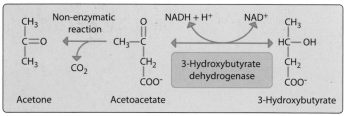

Fig. 3.36.1 Ketone bodies.

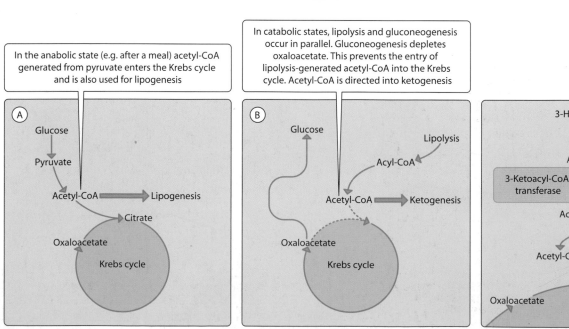

Fig. 3.36.2 Utilization of acetyl-CoA in (A) anabolic and (B) catabolic states.

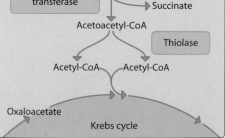

Fig. 3.36.3 Metabolism of ketone bodies.

Regulation of ketogenesis

The principal regulator of ketogenesis is the insulin-to-glucagon ratio. Ketogenesis is stimulated when the ratio is low.

Utilization of ketone bodies

Importantly, the keto acids are also a metabolic fuel and can re-enter energy metabolism (Fig. 3.36.4) by oxidation of hydroxybutyrate to acetoacetate, yielding NADH, followed by activation of acetoacetate by CoA in an exchange with succinyl-CoA (catalysed by 3-ketoacyl-CoA transferase). Subsequently, acetoacetate-CoA is cleaved by thiolase to give two molecules of acetyl-CoA, and these can be oxidized in the Krebs cycle.

Ketone bodies serve as a fuel for the brain and the muscle. Normally, the brain uses approximately 140 g glucose (600 kcal) per day. However, cardiac muscle and renal cortex use acetoacetate in preference to glucose. During prolonged starvation, the brain also adjusts to the use of ketone bodies, which may eventually constitute as much as 75% of its fuel. Since utilization of ketone bodies during starvation limits the need for gluconeogenesis, it spares body proteins.

Ketone bodies and fasting

A moderate ketosis occurs on low-carbohydrate diets taken to reduce weight. There is no evidence that this is harmful. However, massive amount of ketone bodies generated from lipolysis in decompensated diabetes mellitus lead to acidification of extracellular fluid, which is known as the diabetic ketoacidosis.

Table 3.36.1 THE KETOGENIC AMINO ACIDS

Amino acid	Product of amino acid metabolism
Isoleucine	Acetyl CoA
Phenylalanine and tyrosine	Acetoacetate
Lysine and and tryptophan	Acetoacetyl-CoA
Leucine	Hydroxymethylglutaryl-CoA

CONDITIONS LEADING TO ABUNDANT KETONE BODIES

In situations where large amount of acetyl-CoA are formed, any excess not used in the Krebs cycle is converted to ketones. One indication is the smell of acetone on the breath; incidentally, not all people can smell acetone.

Diabetes mellitus

In diabetes, because of the absolute or relative lack of insulin, the excess of anti-insulin hormones activates hormone-sensitive lipase and induces a high rate of lipolysis, generating large amounts of acetyl-CoA. The presence of ketone bodies in the urine or in the blood of a diabetic person is an important warning of impending ketoacidosis.

Diet

A very-low-carbohydrate diet, particularly if accompanied by a high fat intake, will stimulate lipolysis and so generates large amount of acetyl-CoA. This can cause the breath to smell of acetone.

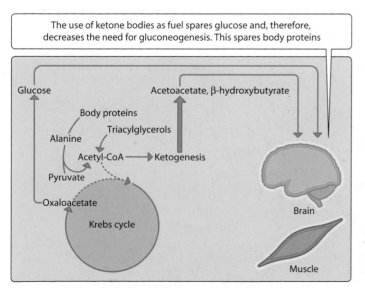

Fig. 3.36.4 Use of ketone bodies as metabolic fuel.

37. Synthesis of fatty acids and lipogenesis

Questions
- How is acetyl-CoA carboxylase regulated?
- How does the fatty acid synthetase complex work?
- Which electron carrier is required by fatty acid synthesis?

Fatty acid synthesis is an anabolic pathway that enables the storage of metabolic fuel in adipose tissue as triacylglycerols (lipogenesis). In the fed state, lipogenesis is closely linked to carbohydrate metabolism. Understanding this is fundamental for nutrition and issues associated with obesity and weight-loss regimens.

Note that, apart from being the main fuel storage, fatty acids are also components of vital structural molecules, such as phospholipids, hormone-like substances, such as prostaglandins, and signalling species, such as inositol phosphates. They also act as signalling molecules themselves.

Synthesis of the fatty acids
Synthesis of fatty acids requires acetyl-CoA (Fig. 3.37.1). The two main stages of the pathway are the carboxylation of acetyl-CoA and the synthesis of the fatty acid chain. The latter takes place on a large multienzyme complex, the **fatty acid synthetase**. Synthesis of fatty acids takes place in the cytoplasm.

Acetyl-CoA carboxylase: the rate limiting step of fatty acid synthesis
Acetyl-CoA carboxylase is a biotin-dependent enzyme that converts C2 acetyl-CoA into C3 malonyl-CoA (Fig. 3.37.2). This reaction is regulated by several mechanisms:

- allosteric interactions: citrate stimulates and palmitoyl-CoA inhibits the enzyme
- phosphorylation/dephosphorylation: phosphorylation inhibits the enzyme and dephosphorylation activates (so it is inhibited by glucagon)
- enzyme synthesis: high-carbohydrate/low-fat intake increases the expression of the enzyme and starvation or high fat/low carbohydrate diet downregulate it.

Fatty acid synthetase
Fatty acid synthetase is a seven-enzyme complex. The complex is a dimer arranged head-to-tail, and it also contains the **acyl-carrier protein**. The sequence of reactions starts with positioning malonyl-CoA and the condensation of a molecule of malonyl-CoA and acetyl-CoA by ketoacyl synthase. Next there is the reduction by NADPH, dehydration and another reduction, yielding an acyl chain elongated by two carbons.

This product immediately enters the next cycle of synthesis: six further cycles are required to produce a 16-carbon molecule of palmitic acid.

The fatty acid synthesized by the synthetase may be elongated further by fatty acid elongase or it may be desaturated (however, human desaturase does not act beyond C10 of the fatty acid chain).

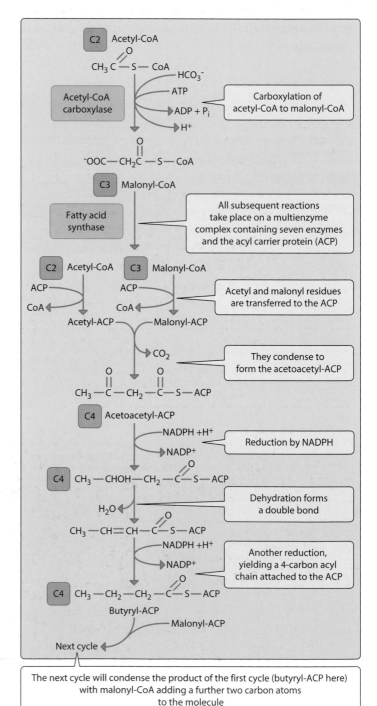

Fig. 3.37.1 Fatty acid synthesis.

Citrate–malate antiport as means of supplying acetyl-CoA to the cytoplasm

For the synthesis of fatty acids to proceed, acetyl-CoA is required in the cytoplasm. There is, however, no transporter for acetyl-CoA from the mitochondria. Instead of direct transport, acetyl-CoA is condensed with oxaloacetate, forming citrate, and it is the citrate that exits mitochondria in exchange for malate. In the cytosol, citrate is cleaved into oxaloacetate and acetyl-CoA. Oxaloacetate is oxidized to malate and may be further converted to pyruvate by the malic enzyme, yielding NADPH. The NADPH thus produced can be used for fatty acid synthesis (another source of NADPH is the pentose phosphate pathway) (see Ch. 30).

Lipogenesis: synthesis of triacylglycerols

Acetyl-CoA molecules are incorporated into triacylglycerols (Fig. 3.37.3), the storage form of neutral fat. In the liver, the source of glycerol phosphate for triacylglycerol synthesis is the glycerol kinase reaction. In the adipose tissue, glycerol phosphate is derived from dihydroxyacetone phosphate: this is another example of how glycolysis favours fat storage.

The role of insulin

Insulin stimulates lipogenesis (see Ch. 53). It is well known that diabetic patients treated with insulin gain weight.

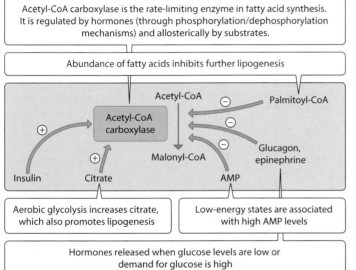

Fig. 3.37.2 Acetyl-CoA carboxylase is the regulatory enzyme of lipogenesis.

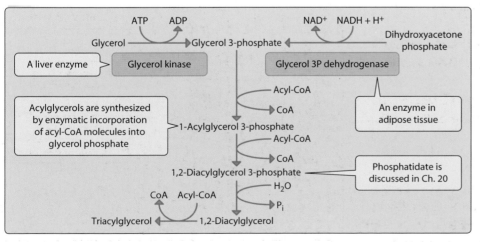

Fig. 3.37.3 The synthesis of triacylglycerols.

38. Key metabolites: pyruvate oxaloacetate and acetyl-CoA

Questions
- Compare the fate of pyruvate during anaerobic and aerobic glycolysis
- Why are anaplerotic reactions yielding oxaloacetate metabolically important?
- What is the biosynthetic role of the acetyl-CoA?

Pyruvate, oxaloacetate and acetyl-CoA are the three metabolites that link different fuel metabolism pathways.

Pyruvate
Pyruvate metabolism (Fig. 3.38.1) depends on the availability of O_2 and the energy state of the cell:

- pyruvate can be oxidized to acetyl-CoA by the pyruvate dehydrogenase complex
- it can be carboxylated to oxaloacetate by pyruvate carboxylase (anaplerotic reaction)
- it can be transaminated to alanine by alanine transaminase
- it can be converted into lactate in anaerobic glycolysis by lactate dehydrogenase
- it can be produced from phosphoenolpyruvate by pyruvate kinase.

Oxaloacetate
Oxaloacetate is formed from malate in the Krebs cycle (Fig. 3.38.2):

- it condenses with acetyl-CoA to form citrate
- it can be generated in the cytoplasm from citrate by the citrate lyase reaction
- it can also be transported out of the mitochondria as malate
- it can be transaminated to aspartate

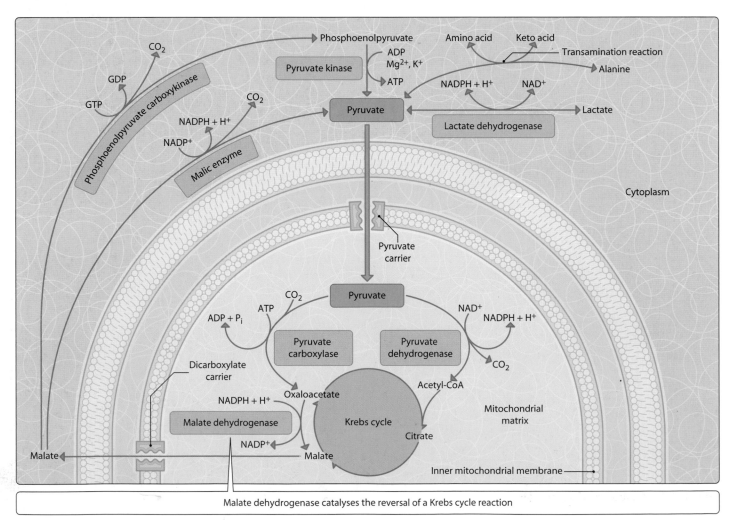

Malate dehydrogenase catalyses the reversal of a Krebs cycle reaction

Fig. 3.38.1 Metabolism of pyruvate.

- it can enter gluconeogenesis by being converted to phospho-enolpyruvate in a reaction catalysed by phosphoenolpyruvate carboxykinase, a key gluconeogenetic enzyme
- it can be formed from pyruvate by pyruvate carboxylase.

Acetyl-CoA

Acetyl-CoA is a 2-carbon compound that links energy and biosynthetic pathways (Fig. 3.38.3):

- it is oxidized to CO_2 in the Krebs cycle
- it is an essential building block of fatty acids

- it is a product of fatty acid oxidation.
- it enters ketogenesis if oxaloacetate supply is poor
- it serves as a biosynthetic precursor of cholesterol and other steroids.

Transport of acetyl-CoA out of the mitochondria for use in biosynthetic pathways is decribed in Ch. 27.

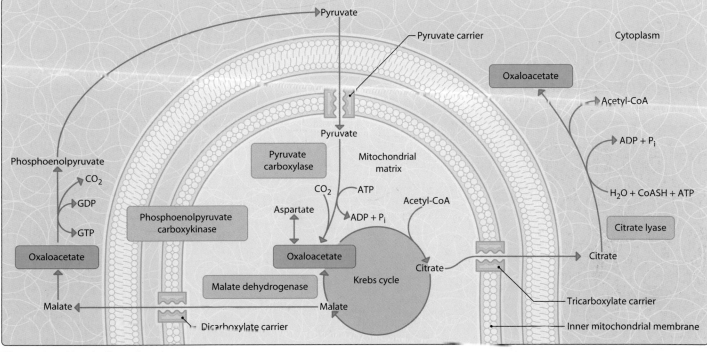

Fig. 3.38.2 Metabolism of oxaloacetate.

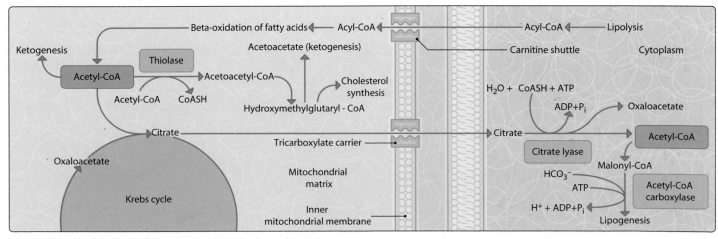

Fig. 3.38.3 Metabolism of acetyl-CoA.

39. Metabolism of amino acids and nitrogen

Questions

- Why is transamination reaction a key reaction in body nitrogen metabolism?
- What mechanism allows the elimination of free ammonia from the body?

Proteins present in the body undergo degradation and resynthesis: they have widely different half-lives. The two issues to consider in the metabolism of the amino acids are:

- the fate of the nitrogen atom
- the fate of the rest of the molecule, the 'carbon skeleton'.

Nitrogen balance

Importantly, proteins are all either structural or functional: there are no specific storage proteins. Amino acids are replenished from dietary protein and any excess is excreted. Nitrogen balance is the difference between the intake and the excretion of nitrogen. If intake is greater than excretion, the nitrogen balance is positive: if excretion exceeds intake, it is negative. Nitrogen excretion can be measured either by direct measurement of urinary nitrogen excretion or, with slight approximation, by measuring urea nitrogen.

The fate of nitrogen

Because nitrogen is toxic to tissues, it needs to be safely excreted. Vertebrates are ureotelic (i.e. excrete nitrogen as urea). Amino groups from different amino acids are transferred to α-ketoglutarate in a transamination reaction (see below), forming **glutamate**. Glutamate may accept still more nitrogen, forming **glutamine**, which is synthesized in an ATP-driven reaction. Glutamine is the main nitrogen transport vehicle. It is present in blood in concentrations higher than other amino acids and serves as nitrogen donor in biosyntheses of other amino acids, nucleotides, amino sugars and NAD^+. Excess glutamine is degraded by glutaminase in liver and kidney. Also, glutamate

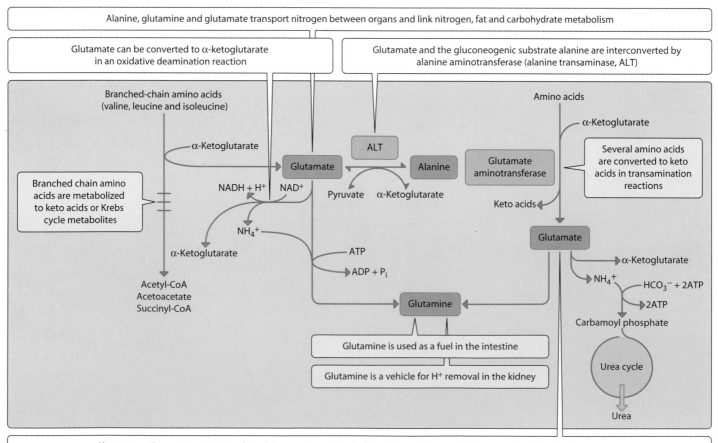

Fig. 3.39.1 Nitrogen metabolism.

and glutamine donate the ammonium ion for the synthesis of **urea**. The overview of nitrogen metabolism is given in Figure 3.39.1.

Transamination

Transamination is carried out by transaminases and involves the transfer of an amino group from an amino acid to a keto acid. It is the key reaction in nitrogen metabolism. The two most important transaminases are **alanine transaminase** (ALT) and **aspartate transaminase** (AST). Both transfer amino groups to α-ketoglutarate (a Krebs cycle metabolite), forming glutamate:

ALT: alanine + α-ketoglutarate $\rightleftharpoons$ pyruvate + glutamate

AST: aspartate + α-ketoglutarate $\rightleftharpoons$ oxaloacetate + glutamate

These are reversible reactions; therefore, glutamate can be used to produce alanine from pyruvate or to yield aspartate for biosyntheses.

The α-keto acids resulting from transamination may either be oxidized or can be converted to glucose. Note that glutamate generated in muscle may be transported to the liver either as glutamine or as alanine (after transamination). In the latter, glutamate is re-formed from alanine in the liver. The prosthetic group of transaminases is pyridoxal phosphate (vitamin B_6).

Glutamate dehydrogenase

Another important reaction in nitrogen metabolism is the reductive amination of α-ketoglutarate. This is a mitochondrial reaction catalysed by glutamate dehydrogenase. Reductive amination fixes the ammonium ion, yielding glutamate.

α-ketoglutarate + NH_4^+ + NADH (NADPH) $\rightleftharpoons$
$$\text{glutamate} + NAD^+ (NADP^+) + H^+$$

The reverse reaction yields α-ketoglutarate and the ammonium ion, which enters the urea cycle. Glutamate dehydrogenase is subject to allosteric regulation. It is inhibited by GTP and ATP and is activated by GDP and ADP. Note that it uses both NAD^+ and $NADP^+$ as coenzymes.

Elimination of the free ammonia

Free ammonia generated in tissues combines with glutamate to form glutamine in the glutamine synthetase reaction. This requires ATP:

$$\text{glutamate} + NH_4^+ + \text{ATP} \rightleftharpoons \text{glutamine} + \text{ADP}$$

Therefore, in mammals, glutamate dehydrogenase and glutamine synthetase are the two enzymes capable of 'fixing' ammonia. Removal of ammonia is important because it is neurotoxic (Ch. 40).

41. Cholesterol and bile acids

Questions
- How is HMG-CoA reductase regulated?
- What is the biological significance of cholesterol?
- How do statin drugs act and what effects do they have on the low density lipoprotein receptor?

Cholesterol is an essential component of cells and is synthesized by most cells. The liver and intestine each produce approximately 10% of total body synthesis. Cholesterol is a key component of membranes, increasing membrane fluidity. It is also a precursor of steroid hormones and vitamin D.

The cholesterol molecule is amphipathic, but in the free form it is virtually insoluble in water. It forms esters with long-chain fatty acids. Free cholesterol and cholesteryl esters are the two forms of cholesterol present in plasma. They are transported between organs as components of lipoproteins (see Ch. 23).

Cholesterol balance
Approximately 700 mg cholesterol is synthesized daily, even if an individual is taking a low-cholesterol diet. An average Western diet contains another 500 mg. The recommendations for low-fat eating suggest intake as low as 200 mg daily.

Cholesterol absorption
Dietary cholesteryl esters are hydrolysed in the intestine by cholesteryl ester hydrolase. The cholesterol is absorbed and incorporated into chylomicrons: 80–90% of cholesterol in plasma remains esterified.

Cholesterol synthesis
Cholesterol is synthesized from acetyl-CoA (Fig. 3.41.1). The rate-limiting step is the reduction of hydroxymethylglutaryl (HMG)-CoA to mevalonate by **HMG-CoA reductase**. Mevalonate is converted to isopentenyl bisphosphate, which is also called an **activated isoprene unit** as it serves as building block for the synthesis of steroid-like molecules. The steroid nucleus comprises six isoprene units (note that altogether there are approximately 5000 known isoprenoids!).

In cholesterol synthesis, six such units condense to form **squalene**. Subsequently, ring closure occurs, and this is followed by several relocations of methyl groups and double bonds, finally yielding cholesterol.

Regulation of cholesterol intake and synthesis
Exogenous cholesterol contained in lipoprotein remnant particles and in low density lipoproteins (LDL) is taken up by cells after these lipoproteins bind to the membrane LDL receptor.

Importantly, dietary cholesterol inhibits hepatic cholesterol synthesis: repressing the HMG-CoA reductase gene. Cholesterol influx also decreases the activity of HMG-CoA synthase, increases the activity of acylCoA:cholesterol acyltransferase (ACAT) and decreases the synthesis of LDL receptor (Fig. 3.41.2).

Cholesterol synthesis is associated with the anabolic state. HMG-CoA reductase activity is increased by insulin and thyroxine and decreased by glucagon and cortisol. Glucagon acts via an ATP-activated protein kinase, which phosphorylates HMG-CoA reductase.

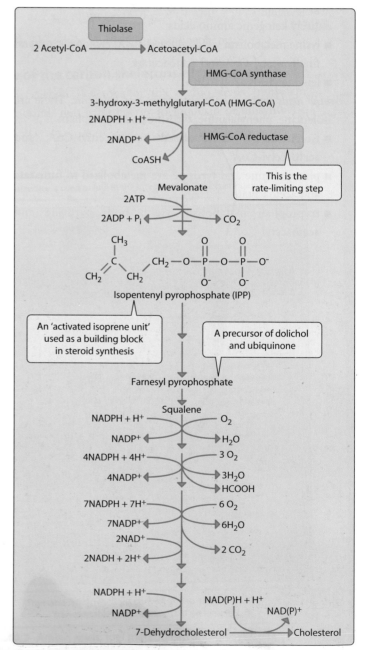

Fig. 3.41.1 Cholesterol synthesis.

The statin drugs, used to combat high cholesterol levels, are competitive inhibitors of HMG-CoA reductase.

Transcription factors in cholesterol synthesis

Lipid metabolism is regulated by a family of transcription factors called the sterol regulatory binding proteins (SREBPs). These bind to the DNA sterol regulatory element. SREBP-2, upregulates enzymes in the cholesterol synthesis pathway, including HMG-CoA reductase and HMG-CoA synthetase.

Biliary excretion of cholesterol: bile acids

The human body cannot degrade the steroid nucleus. Cholesterol is eliminated in bile via the gastrointestinal tract. There is a 3–5 g pool of bile acids that is constantly recirculated; out of this, only 0.3–0.5 g is lost daily in faeces.

Bile contains the primary bile acids, **cholic acid** and **chenodeoxycholic acid**, which are synthesized from cholesterol (Fig. 3.41.3) and free cholesterol. Bile acids enter bile as conjugates with glycine or taurine. In the intestine, secondary bile acids, **deoxycholic acid** and **lithocholic acid** are formed by bacterial action. Lithocholic acid is not absorbed in the intestine.

Bile acids facilitate the absorption of dietary fat, cholesterol and fat-soluble vitamins (Ch. 8).

Regulation of bile acid synthesis

The rate-limiting reaction in bile acid synthesis is catalysed by 7α-hydroxylase. Synthesis of this enzyme is regulated by the nuclear bile acid-binding receptor (farnesoid X receptor), which is a transcription factor (and by bile via a bile acid response element).

Cholesterol increases 7α-hydroxylase activity, and bile acids suppress it. Drainage of bile acids also upregulates HMG-CoA reductase and the LDL receptor. Disruption of 7α-hydroxylase gene results in malabsorption, malnutrition, skin pathologies and eye abnormalities.

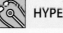 **HYPERCHOLESTEROLAEMIA**

Life style and heredity influence cholesterol balance (a desirable value is <5 mmol/l). Familial hypercholesterolaemia is caused by a mutation in the LDL receptor gene (frequency 1:500 in western countries). A diagnostic feature is tendon xanthoma.

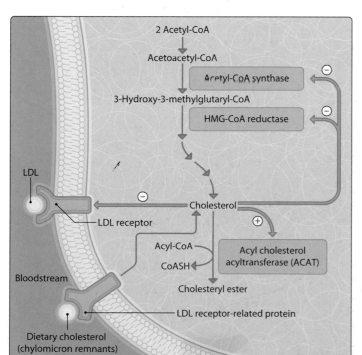

Fig. 3.41.2 Intracellular cholesterol concentration regulates the expression of low density lipoprotein (LDL) receptors and the rate of cholesterol synthesis.

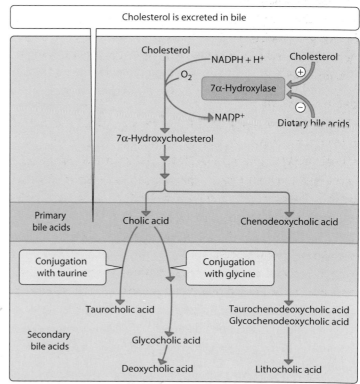

Fig. 3.41.3 Synthesis of bile acids from cholesterol.

42. Haem and bilirubin

Questions
- What is the rate-limiting step in haem synthesis?
- What patterns can be seen for liver function tests in obstructive liver disease?
- What metabolite needs to be measured in a patient with suspected acute intermittent porphyria?

Haem is a metalloporphyrin that incorporates an iron atom (see Fig. 3.15.1). It serves as a prosthetic group for the haemoproteins, oxygen-binding proteins such as haemoglobin, myoglobin, respiratory chain cytochromes, cytochrome P450 and catalase. It is synthesized from the Krebs cycle metabolite succinyl-CoA and is metabolized to bilirubin. The side chains in pyrrole rings possess various combinations of acetyl, propionyl and vinyl residues. These side chains determine porphyrin diversity.

Haem synthesis
In mammals, haem is synthesized from succinyl-CoA and glycine (Fig. 3.42.1). A vitamin, pyridoxal phosphate, participates in this first reaction, and its product is D-aminolaevulinate. Condensation of two molecules of yields prophobilinogen. Subsequently four molecules of porphobilinogen condense: first into a linear tetrapyrrole and then into (type I and type III) uroporphyrinogens. These are decarboxylated to coproporphyrinogens; coproporphyrinogen III is converted into protoporphyrinogen IX, and subsequently into protoporphyrin IX. Finally, ferrochelatase inserts Fe^{2+}, yielding haem.

The haem synthesis pathway weaves between the mitochondria and cytosol. The first reaction and the final steps from coproporphyrin to haem are mitochondrial; other reactions are cytosolic.

Haem degradation
Microsomal haem oxygenase breaks up the tetrapyrrole ring, to form a linear structure, **biliverdin**. At this point, Fe^{2+} is oxidized to Fe^{3+} and released (Fig. 3.42.2). Mammals reduce biliverdin further to **bilirubin**. Bilirubin is non-polar and is transported to the liver bound to albumin (Fig. 3.42.3). Inside hepatocytes, it remains bound to ligandin and protein Y. Glucuronyltransferase conjugates bilirubin with glucuronic acid, which makes it water soluble.

Secretion of bilirubin into the bile involves the multidrug resistance protein 2 (MRP-2), which belongs to the family of ATP-binding cassette transporters (ABC).

In the ileum, bacterial β-glucuronidases remove glucuronides, and bilirubin is converted to urobilinogen. Urobilinogen is also excreted in urine.

Diagnosis of jaundice
Clinical laboratories measure both free (unconjugated) bilirubin and bilirubin glucuronides. The so-called **direct bilirubin test** measures water-soluble bilirubin glucuronides. The **indirect bilirubin test** measures non-polar free bilirubin. Only unconjugated bilirubin crosses the blood–brain barrier. Measurement of bilirubin and some hepatic enzymes is used in the differential diagnosis of jaundice. Three patterns can be observed (Table 3.42.1):

Porphyrias
Porphyrias are rare diseases caused by deficiencies of haem-synthesizing enzymes. A decrease in haem synthesis derepresses D-alanine synthetase and leads to accumulation of metabolites. There are two major classes of porphyria.

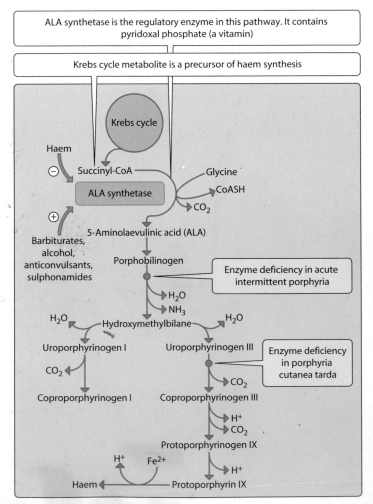

Fig. 3.42.1 Haem synthesis.

Table 3.42.1 LABORATORY DIAGNOSIS OF JAUNDICE

Type	Indirect (unconjugated) bilirubin test	Direct (conjugated) bilirubin test	Transaminases	GGT	AP
Prehepatic (excessive haemolysis)	↑	N	N	N	N
Intrahepatic jaundice	–	↑↑	↑	↑	N
Posthepatic (obstruction)	N	↑	N/↑	↑↑	↑↑

↑, increased; N, normal; GGT, gamma-glutamyltransferase; AP, alkaline phosphatase.

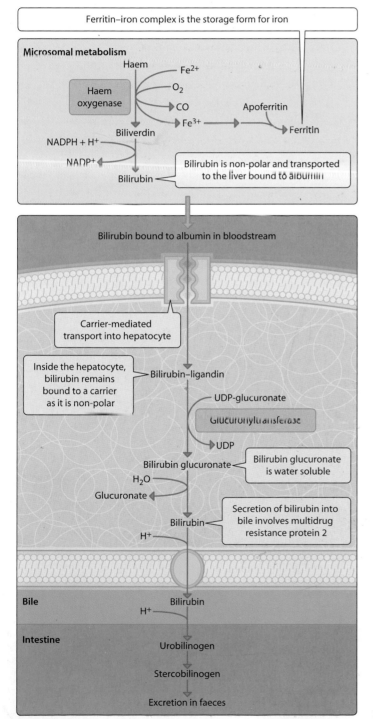

Fig. 3.42.2 Degradation of haem.

Hepatic porphyrias. These can be precipitated by factors that increase hepatic haem synthesis, such as alcohol or drugs (barbiturates or sulphonamides). They lead to neurotoxicity and photosensitivity. Hepatic porphyrias include **acute intermittent porphyria** (porphobilinogen deaminase deficiency) and **porphyria cutanea tarda** (uroporphyrinogen decarboxylase deficiency).

Bone marrow porphyrias. These cause photosensitivity but not neurotoxicity. The most common is **variegate porphyria** (protoporphyrinogen oxidase deficiency)

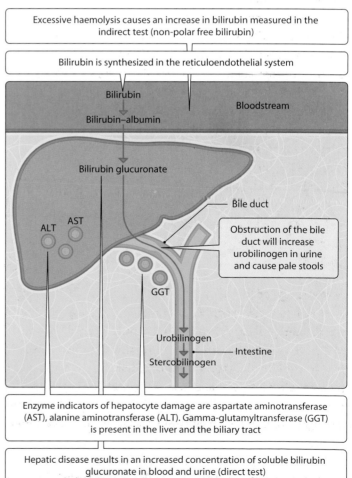

Fig. 3.42.3 Bilirubin transport, metabolism and excretion.

43. Synthesis of amino acids

Questions
- How is tetrahydrofolate involved in amino acid synthesis?
- What is the metabolic defect in phenylketonuria?
- What amino acids can be synthesized from the Krebs cycle metabolites?

While plants and bacteria are able to synthesize all amino acids, mammals are not. Those that they cannot synthesize are known as the essential amino acids. Out of the 20 amino acids that are encoded in the genome, 9 are essential. These are histidine, isoleucine, leucine, lysine, methionine, phenylalanine, threonine, tryptophan and valine.

The other eleven—alanine, arginine, asparagine, aspartate, cysteine, glutamate, glutamine, glycine, proline, serine and tyrosine—can be synthesized (Fig. 3.43.1).

Synthesis of non-essential amino acids
Recall that amino acids are metabolized to energy intermediates. The reverse is also true; most of the non-essential amino acids are generated from either glycolytic or Krebs cycle intermediates.

Glutamate. Reductive amination generates glutamate from the Krebs cycle metabolite α-ketoglutarate (glutamate dehydrogenase) (Ch. 39):

$$\alpha\text{-ketoglutarate} + NAD(P)H + NH_4^+ H^+ \rightleftharpoons glutamate + NAD(P)^+$$

Glutamine and proline. Both are synthesized from glutamate. Proline synthesis requires two reductions by NADH and NADPH. This pathway also yields **ornithine**, which is needed in the urea cycle.

Arginine. Glutamate is also a precursor for arginine, which is synthesized in the urea cycle. Arginine is a precursor for **nitric oxide** and **creatine**.

Alanine. Pyruvate yields alanine in a transamination reaction:

$$pyruvate + glutamate \rightleftharpoons alanine + \alpha\text{-ketoglutarate}$$

Aspartate. Glutamate is transaminated with oxaloacetate to give aspartate, which is itself a substrate for synthesis of **pyrimidines**

$$oxaloacetate + glutamate \rightleftharpoons aspartate + \alpha\text{-ketoglutarate}$$

Asparagine. This is generated from aspartate.

Serine. The glycolytic intermediate 3-phosphoglycerate is used to synthesize serine.

Glycine. Serine and CO_2 participate in the formation of glycine by transmethylation (tetrahydrofolate (THF) participates in this reaction). Glycine is important in the synthesis of nucleotides, creatine, porphyrins and glutathione.

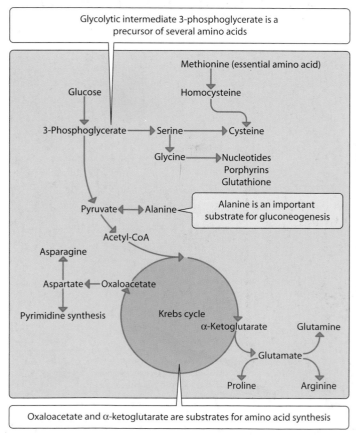

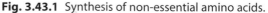

Fig. 3.43.1 Synthesis of non-essential amino acids.

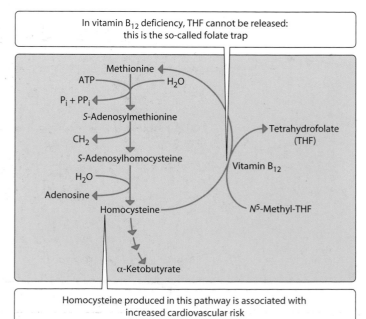

Fig. 3.43.2 The methionine salvage pathway.

Cysteine. Serine and homocysteine (derived from from methionine) participate in cysteine formation. The **methionine salvage pathway** utilizes a vitamin B$_{12}$-catalysed reaction and the 1-carbon carrier THF. Homocysteine produced in this pathway has been associated with increased cardiovascular risk (Fig. 3.43.2; see also Ch. 9).

Tyrosine. This is synthesized from tryptophan (see p. 17).

Essential amino acids

The essential amino acids are synthesized in bacterial or plant cells, also from energy metabolites and pentose phosphate pathway intermediates.

- valine and leucine are synthesized from pyruvate
- tryptophan and phenylalanine from phosphoenolpyruvate and erythrose 4-phosphate
- histidine from ribose 5-phosphate
- methionine, threonine, lysine and isoleucine from oxaloacetate.

The role of amino acids in other biosyntheses

Amino acids participate in several biosynthetic reactions (Fig. 3.43.3):

- nucleotides
- porphyrins
- creatine
- glutathione.

Specialized derivatives of amino acids

Amino acids are a source of specialized products, particularly hormones and neurotransmitters:

- tyrosine is the precursor of DOPA (L-3,4-dihydroxyphenylalanine), dopamine, norepinephrine and epinephrine
- tryptophan is a precursor of serotonin (5-hydroxytryptamine)
- histidine yields histamine
- glutamate is decarboxylated to γ-aminobutyrate (GABA).

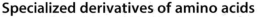 **INBORN ERRORS OF AMINO ACID METABOLISM**

The first described inborn error of metabolism was **phenylketonuria**. It is associated with mental retardation, which can be prevented by dietary restriction of phenylalanine. Screening programmes for newborns use a blood-spot test and the spectrofluorimetric measurement to facilitate early detection of this abnormality. Phenylketonuria results from a deficiency of phenylalanine hydroxylase, which catalyses the hydroxylation of phenylalanine to tyrosine. The disorder, if untreated, leads to mental retardation within few months of birth; this is prevented by the phenylalanine-free diet. The inborn errors of amino acid metabolism cause a wide range of mostly very rare diseases, seen usually in the paediatric departments.

Phenylketonuria is an example of the effectiveness and benefits of early screening. The other one is the screening of newborns for hypothyroidism, which employs the measurement of thyroid-stimulating hormone.

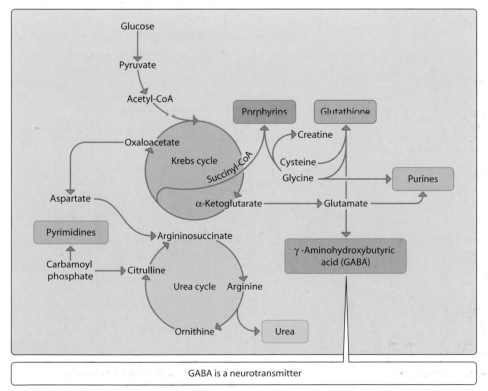

Fig. 3.43.3 Amino acids are precursors of other nitrogen-containing molecules.

44. Purine and pyrimidine metabolism

Questions
- What is the role of nucleotides in activation of substrates?
- What is the rate-limiting step in purine synthesis?
- What is the biological role of the salvage pathways in purine and pyrimidine synthesis?

Purines and pyrimidines are nitrogenous bases (see Ch. 45 for their structures); they are components of DNA, RNA, coenzymes (e.g. NAD^+), high-energy storage molecules (e.g. ATP), activation molecules (e.g. UDP-glucose in glycogen synthesis) and signalling molecules (e.g. cGMP).

The interesting characteristic of their metabolism is that they can be synthesized de novo and be generated by salvage pathways.

Synthesis of purines

Purine synthesis takes place on a molecule of ribose, and the atoms forming the purine ring come from several sources (Fig. 3.44.1). The rate-limiting step is the addition of an amino group from glutamine by **amidophosphoribosyl transferase**, which yields 5-phosphoribosylamine. The following steps construct the skeleton of the imidazole ring and then closure of the ring to give inosine 5′-phosphate (IMP). Inosine can be converted into other nucleotides: AMP is synthesized by amino group transfer from aspartate and GMP is formed by dehydrogenation of inosine to xanthosine 5′-phosphate and amino group transfer from glutamine.

The synthesis of IMP requires 3 molecules of ATP. Adenosine and guanosine nucleotides (AMP, ADP, GMP and GDP) control IMP synthesis, inhibiting PRPP synthase.

Synthesis of pyrimidines

Pyrimidine synthesis takes place in the cytosol. In contrast to the purines, the pyrimidine ring is constructed before the addition of ribose. The atoms in the ring derive from aspartate and carbamoyl phosphate (Fig. 3.44.2). The reaction of carbamoyl phosphate with aspartic acid catalysed by **aspartate carbamoyltransferase** is the rate-limiting step. Ring closure follows, generating dihydroorotic acid. Further steps give uridine 5′-phosphate (UMP). Other pyrimidine bases can be formed from UMP and it is also phosphorylated to UTP: CTP is formed by the reaction of UTP with glutamine in the presence of ATP and TMP is formed by the reduction of UDP by NADPH to dUDP, which is then converted into dUMP; this reacts with tetrahydrofolate to give TMP.

Pyrimidine synthesis is regulated at two steps: carbamoyl phosphate synthase II is inhibited by UTP and purine nucleotides and is activated by PRPP; aspartate carbamoyltransferase is inhibited by CTP and activated by ATP.

Catabolism of purines and pyrimidines

Purines. First, adenosine and AMP are deaminated to inosine and IMP, respectively, and the bases are released from ribose, yielding hypoxanthine, which is oxidized to xanthine

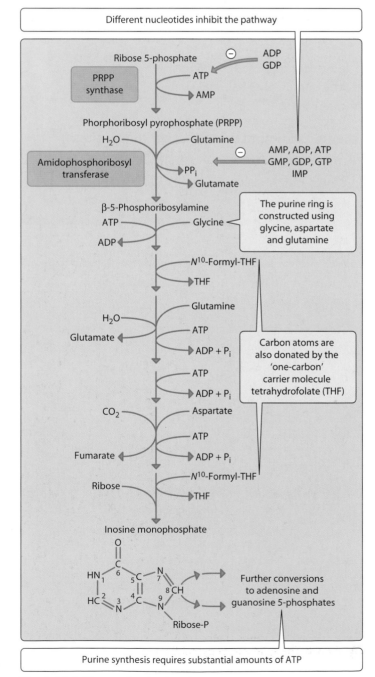

Fig. 3.44.1 The synthesis of purines.

and then to uric acid by the enzyme xanthine oxidase. Guanosine is converted to guanine and then to xanthine.

Pyrimidines. Pyrimidines are first dephosphorylated. Cytidine is oxidatively deaminated to uridine. This is reduced to dihydrouracil by NADPH and the ring is cleaved by hydration. There follows deamination and decarboxylation; this forms β-alanine or β-aminoisobutyrate. Thymine is analogously reduced to dihydrothyronine and yields β-aminoisobutyrate. Aminoisobutyrate can be converted to succinyl-CoA.

Salvage reactions

Salvage reactions reutilize nucleoside bases released during degradation of nucleic acids, thus decreasing the need for de novo synthesis. The free bases can be phosphoribosylated by **phosphoribosyltransferases** using PRPP to form purine 5'-mononucleotides and releasing pyrophosphate (PPi):

$$\text{nucleoside base} + \text{PRPP} \rightarrow \text{NMP} + \text{PPi}$$

where N is any base. Cytosine cannot be salvaged.

Formation of deoxyribonucleotides

Formation of deoxyribonucleotides is accomplished by ribonucleotide reductase:

$$\text{ribonucleotide bisphosphate} + \text{protein(2SH)} \rightleftharpoons$$
$$\text{deoxyribonucleotide bisphosphate} + \text{protein(-S-S-)} + H_2O$$

Ribonucleoside reductase acts on adeninosine, guanine and uridine phosphates and dTMP is formed by the methylation of dUDP. The enzyme is feedback regulated by the concentrations of individual deoxyribonucleotides.

GOUT

Gout is a heterogeneous disease characterized by increased uric acid concentration in plasma. It is also associated with arthritis, renal disease including kidney stones and urate deposits in tissues (tophi). It can be caused by either increased production or (most cases) decreased renal excretion of uric acid.

LESH–NYHAN SYNDROME

Lesh–Nyhan syndrome is a very rare X-linked deficiency of hypoxanthine phosphoribosyltransferase. It is characterized by psychomotor retardation and, characteristically, self-mutilation. Very high uric acid levels are observed.

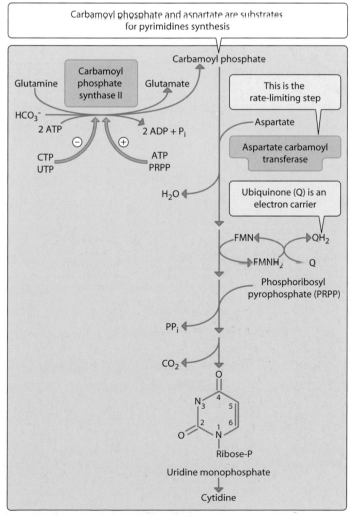

Fig. 3.44.2 The synthesis of pyrimidines.

45. DNA and RNA

Questions
- What are the 'building blocks' of DNA and RNA?
- What bonds and interactions are important in maintaining DNA structure?
- What is the proteome?

Genome and proteome

The genome is the entire set of genes present in an organism. The proteome is the entire set of proteins.

The polymers of nucleotides, deoxyribonucleic acid (DNA) and ribonucleic acid (RNA), constitute the chemical basis of heredity. The central dogma of molecular biology is that the information coded in DNA is translated through RNA into structural and functional proteins.

The basic units of nucleic acids
Definitions

Nucleosides are purine or pyrimidine bases (Fig. 3.45.1) linked to ribose or 2′-deoxyribose (Fig. 3.45.2).

Nucleotides are phosphorylated nucleosides (usually on the 5′-position of the sugar).

Nucleoside monophosphates are nucleotides with phosphoryl group esterified to the hydroxyl of the sugar (3′ and 5′, but most are 5′). Nucleoside di- and triphosphates have additional one or two phosphate groups attached, respectively.

Purines are adenine (A) and guanine (G); both are present in DNA and RNA.

Pyrimidines are cytosine (C), thymine (T) and uracil (U); cytosine occurs in both DNA and RNA but DNA contains thymine and RNA contains uracil (Fig. 3.44.2).

Pentose sugar in nucleosides is supplied by the pentose phosphate pathway.

Gene

A gene has been defined as a sequence of DNA bases coding for one protein (one gene–one protein). However, genes may overlap and a given DNA sequence can be a part of different peptides. Therefore the one gene–one polypeptide principle is more accurate. Genes reside at defined places (loci) in the DNA molecule. There are between 30 000 and 40 000 genes in the human genome. However, the 'overlap' and resulting alternative splicing enables many more proteins to be coded in the DNA. The DNA in eukaryotes is not continuous linked genes: it consists of **exons** (coding sequences) and **introns** (non-coding sequences).

Nucleic acid structures
DNA

DNA is a duplex structure. It is composed of two complementary strands, each being a polymer of nucleotides. Each strand contains nitrogenous bases linked by the β-N-glycosidic bond to the C1 of deoxyribose. A nucleotide is a nucleoside (base plus

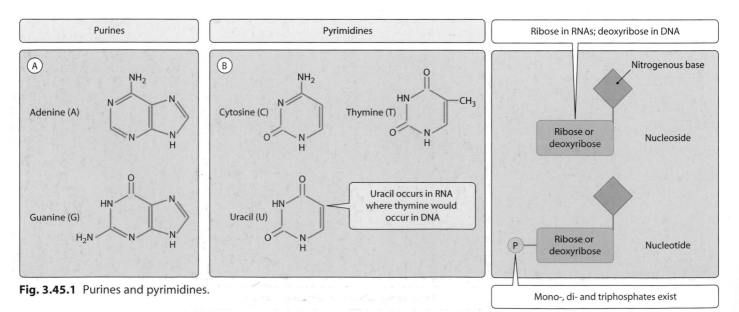

Fig. 3.45.1 Purines and pyrimidines.

Fig. 3.45.2 Nucleosides and nucleotides.

sugar) esterified with phosphate (usually at C5 of the sugar). Phosphodiester bonds link sugar molecules in a nucleic acid, joining carbon 5′ to 3′. Conventionally, the sequence of bases in a nucleic acid is written from the 5′-end (where there is a free phosphate group) to the 3′-end (a free hydroxyl group) (Fig. 3.45.3A).

The secondary structure of a nucleic acid is the double helix, which contains 10 bases per turn and repeats every 34 Å (3.4 nm). The helix is stabilized by hydrogen bonds between the complementary bases A–T and G–C (Fig. 3.45.3B). Similarly to proteins, hydrophobic interactions and van der Waals forces play an important role in determining the secondary structure. Consequently, hydrophobic parts of nucleic acid components are 'buried' within the helix, and the polar parts are exposed to the outside. The fact that the double helix is held together by weak interactions rather than covalent bonds facilitates winding and unwinding of the structure.

The DNA helix in its B and A forms has two grooves (a major and a minor groove), which provide access to the interior of the molecule. This is important for DNA-binding proteins such as transcription factors. The DNA is packed into chromosomes: 22 pairs of autosomes and a pair of sex chromosomes.

RNA

There are several types of RNA:

- mRNAs, which participate in transcription, acting as the messenger links from DNA to protein synthesis; mRNA transcribed from coding regions of the DNA is known as transcriptome
- transfer RNAs (tRNAs), which transport specific amino acids to the place of polypeptide chain synthesis on the ribosome
- ribosomal RNAs (rRNAs), which form structural parts of the ribosome
- small nucleolar RNAs (snoRNAs), which play a role in modifying rRNA
- micro RNAs (mi RNAs) and short interfering RNAs (si RNAs), which contribute to the regulation of gene expression.

The set of nitrogenous bases constituting RNA differs from DNA in that thymine (T) is substituted by uracil (U). The structure of RNA follows the same general principles as DNA. However, different types of RNA include both single-stranded molecules, such as mRNA, and ones with mixed helical and single-stranded regions (tRNA).

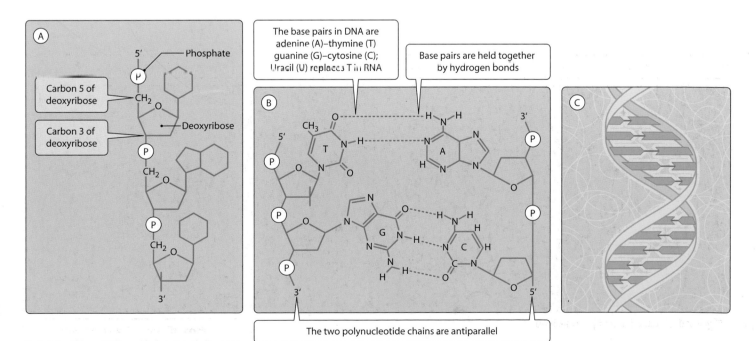

Fig. 3.45.3 The structure of DNA.

46. Replication and transcription of nucleic acids

Questions
- What is of interest about mitochondrial DNA?
- What is 'reverse transcription'?

The semiconservative replication (Fig. 3.46.1) of a nucleic acid (DNA in mammals and RNA in viruses) provides genome continuity through generations. The processes of **transcription** and **translation** convert the DNA information contained in the base sequence of DNA (genome) into the set of protein molecules (proteome) (Fig. 3.46.2).

Incidentally, the notion of unidirectional flow of information from DNA to RNA is not entirely accurate. Retroviruses, which carry their genome as RNA, have the means for reverse transcription; this means that they can write the information contained in their RNA into DNA to incorporate into the host DNA.

As the sequence of DNA bases encodes both exons (coding sequences) and introns (non-coding sequences), the messenger RNA (mRNA) formed by transcription has to be modified. The introns are excised and the exons spliced together (Fig. 3.46.2). Apart from nuclear DNA, genomes also exist in organelles, in particular in the mitochondria. However, in eukaryotes the mitochondrial DNA constitutes less than 1% of the total DNA. Because the embryo receives its mitochondria from the egg only, mitochondrial DNA is inherited only from the mother.

DNA replication

DNA replication is the means of maintaining genetic information through generations. It is initiated at the start of the S phase of the cell cycle. **DNA polymerase** replicates the DNA in a semiconservative manner adding nucleotides at the 3′-end. The **leading** strand is synthesized continuously in the 5′ to 3′ direction. However, the other (**lagging**) strand is constructed as short fragments (**Okazaki fragments**) synthesized also 5′ to 3′ but in the 'backward' direction. Okazaki fragments are then linked by a **ligase**. Replication requires a 3′ priming end to start: this is usually provided by RNA. There are several DNA polymerases: one usually drives replication, and others are involved in DNA repair, which also involves exonuclease activity.

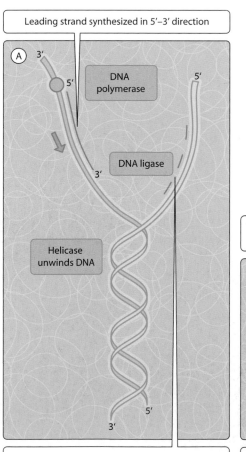

Leading strand synthesized in 5′–3′ direction

(A) 3′

5′

DNA polymerase

5′

DNA ligase

3′

Helicase unwinds DNA

5′

3′

Lagging strand synthesized as fragments (Okazaki fragments) later linked by DNA ligase

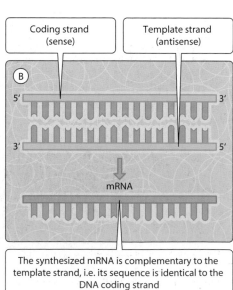

Coding strand (sense)

Template strand (antisense)

(B)

5′   3′

3′   5′

mRNA

The synthesized mRNA is complementary to the template strand, i.e. its sequence is identical to the DNA coding strand

Fig. 3.46.1 Semiconservative DNA replication and formation of mRNA.

Transcription

Transcription is a prelude to protein synthesis. The single-stranded mRNA sequence copies the information contained in DNA and provides a physical template for protein synthesis.

DNA contains the coding (**sense**) strand and the template (**antisense**) strand. The synthesis of mRNA takes place on the antisense strand so that the sequence of bases of the formed mRNA is identical to the coding strand.

Synthesis of mRNA is by **RNA polymerase** and the formed mRNAs vary in size between 500 and 10 000 base pairs. Transcription proceeds from the 5′- to the 3′-end of a gene. Base sequences located before the start point of transcription (i.e. the 5′ end) are referred to as upstream and those lying in the 3′ direction from the start point as downstream. The transcription start point is surrounded by the **promoter**: a sequence of DNA required for the RNA polymerase to bind to the template strand. At the end of each gene, there is a terminating sequence that causes the dissociation of RNA polymerase. During transcription, the section of DNA attached to RNA polymerase separates into a single strand. As the RNA polymerase moves along the

DNA, the 3′-hydroxyl group of each last nucleotide in the growing mRNA reacts with 5′-nucleoside triphosphate. Pyrophosphate is released, and the phosphodiester bond is formed.

The newly synthesized RNA needs to be further processed. This involves capping the 5′-end to provide stability and to facilitate its binding to ribosomes. The introns are spliced out and a polyA tail is added at the 3′-end.

Alternative splicing means that different exons can be joined in various combinations to produce mRNA. This increases the number of proteins that may be synthesized from the same strand of DNA. Further, RNA editing occurs, and this allows new bases to be introduced into mRNA sequence after transcription.

The complementarity of binding between DNA strands has been exploited in the development of molecular biology techniques such as DNA cloning (i.e. replication after insertion of DNA fragments into a plasmid or a virus) or replication without cells (using the polymerase chain reaction). The reader should consult textbooks of molecular biology for details.

Fig. 3.46.2 Transcription and translation.

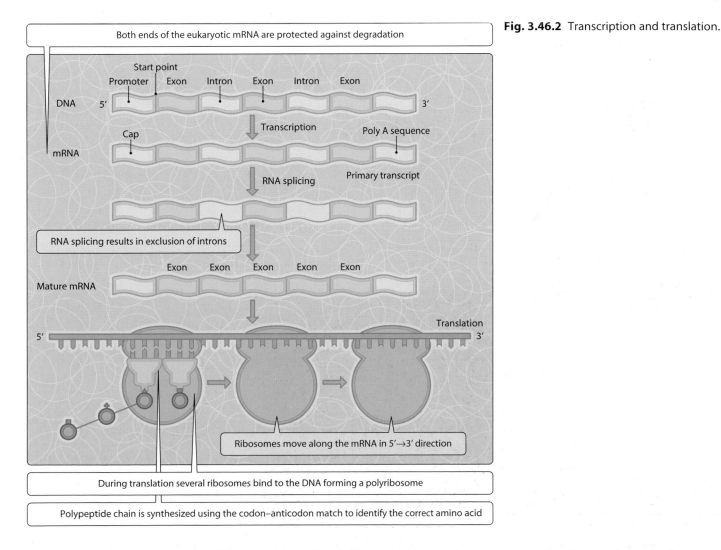

47. Protein synthesis I: the synthetic framework

Questions
- How does tRNA link amino acids to the correct codon?
- How is the framework for protein synthesis assembled?

The synthesis of proteins is controlled by genes, and proteins provide the framework for tissue structure, catalytic molecules and the regulatory/signalling compounds. During protein synthesis, the information contained in the mRNA molecule is converted into the sequence of amino acids in a peptide chain.

Ribosomes
Protein synthesis takes place on ribosomes, organelles located in eukaryotes in the cytoplasm. Ribosomes possess two subunits: a large 50–60S subunit and a small 30–40S subunit (the 'S' reflects their sedimentation rates) (Fig. 3.47.1). They contain RNA (ribosomal or rRNA) and proteins. Ribosomes need to form a complex with mRNA to provide the framework upon which the polypeptide chain can be elaborated (Fig. 3.47.2). The ribosome provides the spatial framework for positioning amino acids bound to tRNA (aminoacyl-tRNA) and the mRNA in a way that facilitates formation of peptide bonds

Earlier, during transcription, the information contained in the molecule of DNA was transferred to mRNA, the sequence of which is identical to that of the DNA coding strand. The binding of a ribosome to mRNA and the formation of the long chain of amino acids in a newly synthesized polypeptide, based on the linear sequence in mRNA, is called **translation**.

Amino acid activation: tRNA
The tRNAs bring amino acids to the site of polypeptide chain synthesis (Fig. 3.47.3). To do this, each tRNA needs to bind a particular amino acid, forming an aminoacyl-RNA. The tRNA molecule is small (74–95 base pairs) with a clover-leaf, three-loop structure held together by the hydrogen bonds between unpaired bases. One of the loops bears the **anticodon**: a triplet of bases complementary to the mRNA base triplet, the **codon**. A particular RNA can bind only one amino acid. However, there is redundancy in the genetic code and, therefore, an amino acid may be activated by more than one tRNA molecule. Codon and anticodon sequences bind through the hydrogen bonds.

An amino acid is linked to the tRNA by an ester bond between its carboxyl group and the hydroxyl group at position 2′ or 3′ in the ribose molecule, which is the 3′-terminal base in the RNA (Fig. 3.47.2). Linking an amino acid with tRNA is catalysed by an **aminoacyl-RNA synthetase**. There are at least 20 aminoacyl-RNA synthetases and each is specific for a particular tRNA–amino acid pair. The synthesis of aminoacyl-tRNA requires ATP. The aminoacyl-RNA synthetase is also capable of proofreading (i.e. it can hydrolyse the 'wrong' aminoacyl-tRNA).

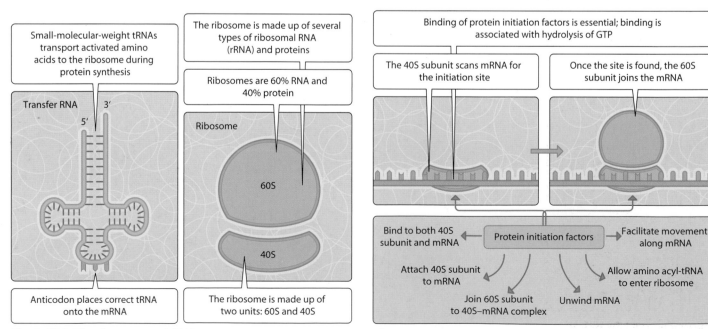

Fig. 3.47.1 The ribosome and tRNA.

Fig. 3.47.2 Formation of a mRNA–ribosome complex.

Mutations

Polymorphisms and mutations are the basis of genetic diversity. Polymorphism is an allele present in at least 1% of the population, and it usually does not affect survival. A mutation is a change in DNA sequence, which usually has a harmful effect. Mutations most often cause loss of function, but gain in function may also occur, and this is important in the development of cancer.

Several kinds of mutation occur. Point mutations are substitutions of a single nucleotide in the DNA sequence. Splice mutations prevent intron splicing and, therefore, the transcribed mRNA is longer than 'normal'. Shifts in reading frame occur after insertion or deletion of a number of bases other than a multiple of three. Such mutations may change the entire amino acid sequence of a protein. They often lead to the early presence of the stop codon and, therefore, result in the synthesis of a shorter protein with abnormal sequence.

Expression of a gene may also be modified by changes other than change in DNA sequence. Such changes include methylation of cytosine residues (by DNA methyltransferases), which change gene transcription by impairing the binding of transcription factors, and alterations in the structure of DNA-associated proteins.

Finally, gene expression may be affected by changes in proteins associated with the DNA. Histones are octameric proteins around which the DNA wraps, forming the so-called **nucleosomes**. Histones can also be modified by methylation, phosphorylation or acetylation, and these changes (particularly acetylation) alter gene transcription.

DNA repair

DNA undergoes constant damage, which may be caused by ionizing radiation or alkylating or deaminating chemicals. Also, errors may occur during DNA replication. DNA repair systems exist to preserve the constancy of the genome. The most common way of repairing damaged DNA is the so-called excision repair mechanism. The damaged section of DNA is excised by endonucleases, and the fragment is resynthesized by DNA polymerase. Some broken phosphodiester bonds (nicks) can be linked back by a ligase enzyme. This is known as direct repair. Alkyl groups can also be enzymatically removed from bases.

Errors of replication are repaired after the new mismatched fragments are recognized by specific proteins on the basis of their degree of methylation (the newly synthesized DNA strand is methylated to a lesser degree than the template strand). Repair includes recognition and binding of repair proteins to the damaged fragment, unwinding by helicase and then excision and resynthesis.

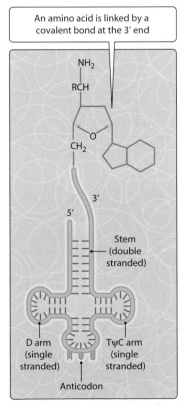

Fig. 3.47.3 The structure of aminoacyl-tRNA.

48. Protein synthesis II: the synthetic process

Questions
- What is meant by saying that there is redundancy in the genetic code?
- What are the three centres relevant to protein synthesis on a ribosome?

Protein synthesis (Fig. 3.48.1) involves mRNA, the aminoacyl-tRNAs and several protein accessory factors brought together on the ribosome. During translation many ribosomes bind to one RNA strand, forming a polyribosome. The anticodon in the aminoacyl-tRNA determines the placement of the amino acid in the sequence determined by the DNA genetic code. There are three active centres on the ribosome, and each has a specific function in protein synthesis:

- **P site** binds the growing peptidyl-tRNA
- **A site** binds the aminoacyl-tRNA
- **E site** is the site through which the released tRNA exits.

There are three stages in protein synthesis: **initiation**, **elongation** and **termination**.

Initiation
At the beginning of the process of protein synthesis, the small subunit of the ribosome associates with the mRNA. Once the initiation sequence on the mRNA is located, the large subunit also binds to the mRNA (see Fig. 3.47.2). Initiation of protein synthesis involves participation of several initiation factors (such as initiation factors IF1, IF2 and IF3 in bacteria) that are necessary for the entry of tRNA into the ribosome and for its binding to mRNA. Different initiation factors operate in bacteria and in mammals. The initiation factor places the **initiator codon** of RNA in what then becomes the P site. Protein synthesis is initiated with methionine, coded by AUG (or GUG). In bacteria, the initiator amino acid is methylated by N^{10}-formyltetrahydrofolate, forming N-formylmethionyl-tRNA. The formyl group is later removed, and in about half of the cases, the methionine is also removed.

Elongation
Elongation of the peptide chain requires accessory elongation factors. The peptide chain transfer takes place on the 60S sub-unit; this subunit has peptidyl transferase activity, which, most interestingly, is associated not with the enzyme but with rRNA (peptidyl transferase is a **ribozyme**). Peptide bond formation requires the hydrolysis of GTP followed by binding of an elongation factor to GDP. Elongation factors (complexed with GTP) participate in the movements of molecules between active sites on the ribosome. Elongation factors are controlled by phosphorylation–dephosphorylation. Some initiation and elongation factors are in fact G-proteins. The sequence of events during elongation is as follows.

1. The new aminoacyl RNA binds to the A site of the ribosome and the peptidyl RNA sits at the P site
2. The peptidyl chain is transferred from the P site RNA to the A site, where it is extended by linking to the aminoacyl-tRNA. The A site now has a peptidyl chain attached that is one amino acid longer than before.
3. The ribosome then moves one triplet of bases further along the mRNA (this is called translocation). Translocation releases the deacylated tRNA through the E site and moves the peptidyl chain to the P site.
4. A new aminoacyl tRNA binds to the A site and the cycle starts again.

Termination
There are 61 base triplets coding for the 20 amino acids; in addition, there are three **termination codons**: UAA, UAG and UGA. When termination codons are encountered by the ribosome, no amino acids are added. Instead, the new protein is released from the mRNA. Termination codons are recognized by release factors. In the termination reaction, the ribosome hydrolyses the peptidyl-tRNA, releasing the new peptidyl chain.

Energy requirements for protein synthesis
Protein synthesis requires much energy. ATP is required for activating amino acids and for unwinding mRNA. GTP hydrolysis provides energy for elongation and termination. The energy for the movement of the ribosome along mRNA comes from hydrolysis of ATP.

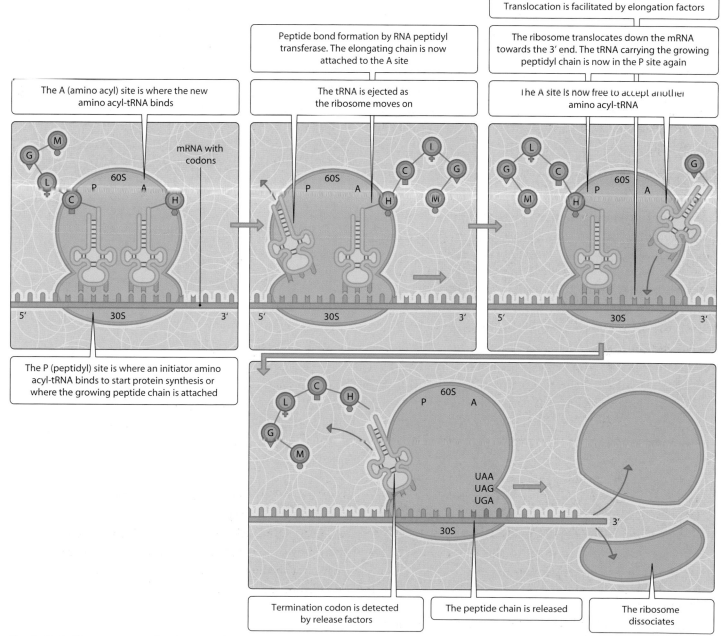

Fig. 3.48.1 The sequence of protein synthesis.

49. Gene expression

Questions
- What is the difference between a promoter and an enhancer?
- What is the mechanisms of activation of transcription factors?
- Give examples of hormonal regulation of gene expression

Promoters and enhancers
Promoters are DNA sequences that direct RNA polymerase to the transcription initiation site. Regulatory proteins (transcription factors) bind to sequences near promoter sites and interact with RNA polymerase. Enhancer sequences play a role similar to promoters but they act further away from the transcription unit (Fig. 3.49.1).

Transcription factors
Transcriptional regulators are mostly DNA-binding proteins that recognize short sequences of DNA, binding to DNA-response elements through characteristic structures (e.g. helix-turn-helix, zinc finger, helix-loop-helix, leucine zipper domains).

Transcription factors are usually small molecules. One factor may be involved in the regulation of many genes (Fig. 3.49.2). They can be *cis* acting (affecting the same gene) or *trans* acting (affecting other genes). Activators either enhance binding of RNA polymerase to the promoter or increase the frequency of transcription (Fig. 3.49.3). Different genes may share promoter or enhancer elements.

Ligand-activated transcription factors are inactive until binding another molecule (Fig. 3.49.4). Transcription factors may also be activated by phosphorylation or inactivated by an inhibitor. For instance NFκB, involved in the immune response, is normally inactivated by an inhibitor protein IκB.

The response elements may form repeat sequences separated by variable numbers of bases. These sequences may bind dimers of the same transcription factor (**homodimer**) or a combination of two factors (**heterodimer**). This provides means for the interaction of different transcription factors to activate one gene (e.g. the 9-*cis*-retinoic acid receptor forms both homo- and heterodimers with other receptors such as thyroid hormone, vitamin D and retinoic acid receptor).

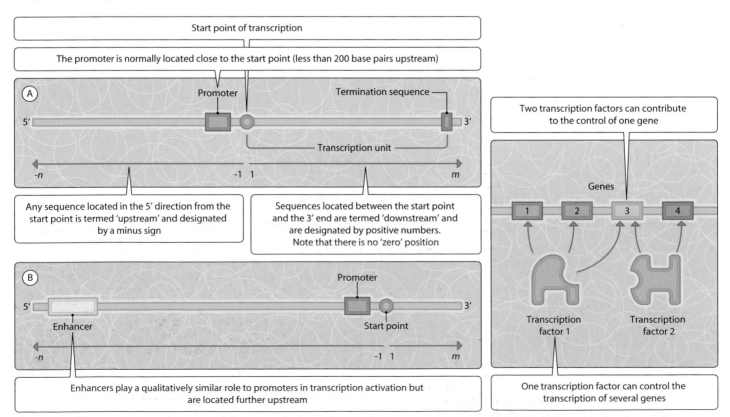

Fig. 3.49.1 The promoter, enhancer and the transcription unit.

Fig. 3.49.2 Transcription factors form a complex regulatory network.

Hormone-response elements

A response element is a DNA sequence that causes a gene to respond to a transcription factor; they are usually located a short distance upstream of the transcription start point. The steroid hormone–receptor complex forms in the cytoplasm and transfers to the nucleus where it binds to the hormone-response element in the promoter of the target gene (Ch. 11).

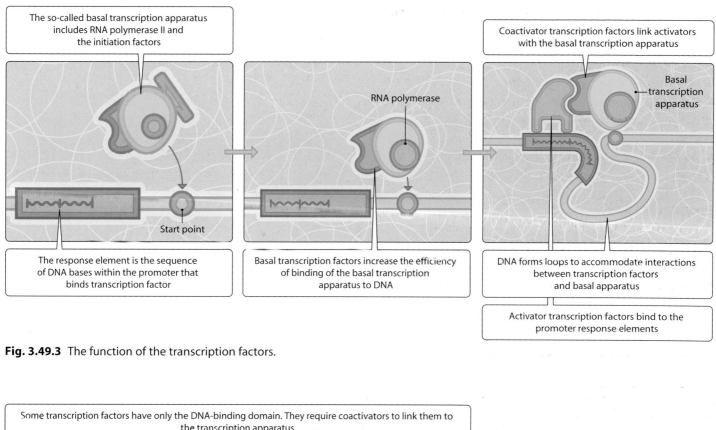

Fig. 3.49.3 The function of the transcription factors.

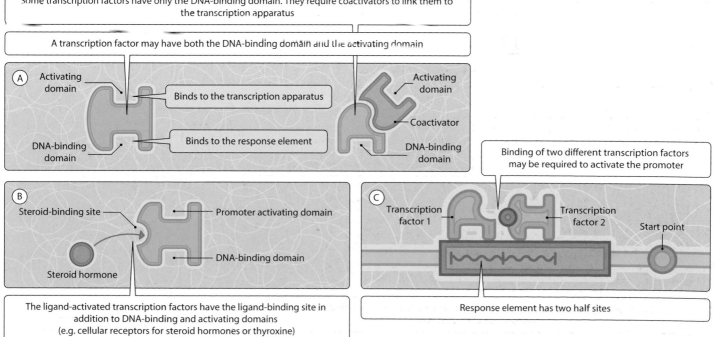

Fig. 3.49.4 The functional domains of transcription factors.

50. Nutrients and diet

Questions
- What are the essential fatty acids?
- How is alcohol metabolized?
- How can one assess nutritional status in a patient?

The main classes of nutrient are shown in Fig. 3.50.1.

Nutrients

Carbohydrates. Dietary carbohydrates include simple sugars, such as sucrose and complex carbohydrates, such as starch. Fibre includes indigestible carbohydrates such as cellulose, hemicellulose, lignin and pectin.

Amino acids. Animal and plant proteins provide the amino acids required by the body. Increased demand for amino acids (dietary protein) is associated with pregnancy, lactation and the adolescent growth spurt.

Fats. Meat, butter, margarines and vegetable oils provide fats (Ch. 20):
- saturated fats (e.g. palmitic acid): animal fats are highly saturated but saturated fats are also present in vegetable oils such as palm oil and cocoa butter
- monounsaturated fatty acids: present in all animal and vegetable fats
- polyunsaturated fatty acids: the ω-6 acids, arachidonic acid (20:4, Δ5,8,11,14) and linoleic acid (18:2, Δ9,12), are present in vegetable seed oils (soybean, canola) and in fish oils; the ω-3 fatty acids are linolenic (18:3, Δ9,12,15), eicosapentaenoic (20:5, Δ5,8,11,14,17) and docosahexaenoic (22:6, Δ4,7,10,13,16,19) and are found in fish and shellfish, and also in some vegetable oils (see Ch. 20 for structures).

Essential nutrients
Essential nutrients cannot be synthesized in the human body and need to be supplied in the diet. They include amino acids, fatty acids and some vitamins and trace elements. Carbohydrates are not essential nutrients.

Essential amino acids: phenylalanine; the branched-chain amino acids valine, leucine and isoleucine; threonine; and methionine and lysine (histidine and arginine are essential for some animals).

Essential lipids. The essential fatty acids (EFA) are linoleic acid and α-linolenic acid (18:3, n-3). Arachidonic acid, eicosapentaenoic acid and docosahexaenoic acid can be made in limited amounts from EFA; however, they may become essential when EFA intake is poor.

Water and minerals. Major minerals are sodium, potassium, chloride, calcium, phosphate and magnesium. Potassium is contained in vegetables and fruit, particularly bananas, and in fruit juices. Calcium is present in milk and milk products, and in some vegetables. Sodium, like phosphate, is widely present in plant and animal cells.

Trace metals and vitamins. See Ch. 8.

Diet and metabolism
The main metabolic fuels are glucose and fatty acids (Figs 3.50.2 and 3.50.3). During prolonged fasting and starvation, proteins are utilized to produce glucose through gluconeogenesis. Fatty acids cannot be converted into glucose, but glycerol is a gluconeogenic substrate. Therefore, lipolysis promotes gluconeogenesis. Ketone bodies are fuel for skeletal and cardiac muscle and become a substitute fuel for the brain during prolonged starvation.

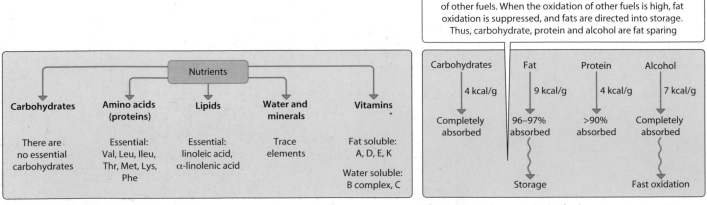

Fig. 3.50.1 Nutrients.

Fig. 3.50.2 The metabolic fuels.

Alcohol

Alcohol is a high-yield metabolic fuel (7 kcal/g). Ethanol is metabolized by cytoplasmic alcohol dehydrogenase (Fig. 3.50.4). High cytoplasmic concentrations of NADH prevent conversion of lactate to pyruvate and inhibit gluconeogenesis. Therefore, alcohol excess may cause hypoglycaemia, because of inadequate endogenous glucose production. NADH also inhibits isocitrate dehydrogenase and α-ketoglutarate dehydrogenase, channelling acetyl-CoA ketogenesis. Further, NADH inhibits fatty acid oxidation, and this stimulates fatty acid synthesis.

Alcohol is also metabolized by the ethanol-inducible microsomal ethanol-oxidizing system (MEOS), which generates acetaldehyde and acetate and uses NADPH. Since the reaction involves molecular O_2, it also generates reactive oxygen species. Acetate is converted in the mitochondria into acetyl-CoA by thiokinase; excess acetyl-CoA leads to ketosis. Prolonged alcohol abuse leads to dyslipidaemia (presenting predominantly as an increase in plasma triacylglycerols).

Nutrients and gene expression

Nutrients affect gene expression. For instance, the activities of key hepatic enzymes in glycolysis, gluconeogenesis, lipolysis and lipogenesis differ in persons remaining on a long-term high-fat diet compared with a high-carbohydrate diet. Further, the amount of dietary cholesterol affects the activity of hydroxy-methylglutaryl (HMG)-CoA reductase, the rate-limiting step in cholesterol synthesis. The peroxisome proliferator-activator receptor is a transcription factor that modulates genes involved in fuel metabolism.

Metabolism at rest

The basal metabolic rate (BMR) is the rate of energy utilization at rest in a thermoneutral environment. It is expressed in kilocalories or kilojoules (1 kcal/mol = 4.19 kJ/mol). It is measured 12 hours after a meal and at body temperature. The BMR in such a thermoneutral environment will reflect energy utilization for respiration, circulation, ion transport across membranes and cellular repair.

The **caloric balance** is the difference between the caloric content of the diet and the energy expenditure. Positive caloric balance leads to weight gain, and negative balance to weight loss. Caloric intake and the level of exercise are the two most important factors determining body weight.

Assessment of nutritional status

The key points in the nutritional assessment are the present clinical status of the patient (anabolic or catabolic), the body mass index (BMI) and the history of weight loss. Nutritional assessment tools attempt to integrate these factors into a score that is then used to assess the need for nutritional support.

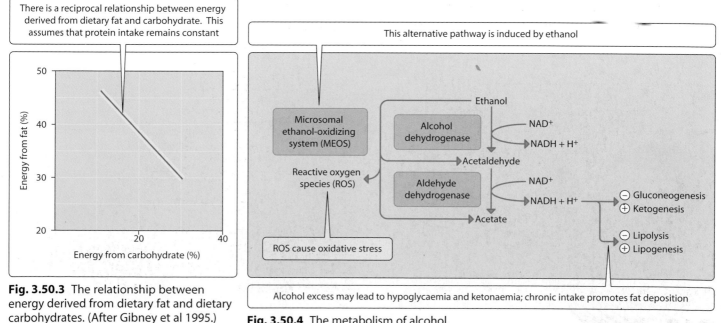

Fig. 3.50.3 The relationship between energy derived from dietary fat and dietary carbohydrates. (After Gibney et al 1995.)

Fig. 3.50.4 The metabolism of alcohol.

51. The fed and fasting states

Questions
- Which metabolic effects in the fed state are the consequence of insulin action?
- In which tissues is most of the body glucose metabolized?
- How would you perform an oral glucose tolerance test?

The fed state is an anabolic state that directs metabolism towards energy storage and synthetic reactions. A carbohydrate-rich meal stimulates the release of insulin, which increases the insulin-to-glucagon ratio (Fig. 3.51.1). This has a number of effects:

- glucose uptake is stimulated in insulin-dependent tissues, principally muscle
- glycogen synthesis increases in liver and muscle
- glucose oxidation is stimulated and gluconeogenesis inhibited
- lipolysis is suppressed and lipogenesis is activated
- in adipose tissue and liver, excess available glucose is directed into the pentose phosphate pathway to provide NADPH for cytoplasmic lipogenesis and other biosynthetic reactions.

Fat is transported from the gut to liver and the peripheral tissues by chylomicrons. Insulin induces lipoprotein lipase, which facilitates hydrolysis of chylomicron triacylglycerols. Glycerol for the synthesis of triacylglycerols comes from glycolysis (dihydroxyacetone phosphate being reduced to glycerol 3-phosphate). Protein synthesis is also stimulated by insulin.

The fasting state
Fasting is a catabolic state that directs metabolism towards the usage of energy stores. During fasting, the insulin-to-glucagon ratio successively decreases (Fig. 3.51.2), resulting in:

- decreased tissue glucose uptake by insulin-dependent tissues (muscle and adipose tissue)
- decreased glycogen synthesis
- increased glycogenolysis and gluconeogenesis
- decreased glucose uptake by muscle and adipose tissue (only 20% of glucose uptake)
- increased proteolysis in muscle
- increased lipolysis generating free fatty acids and providing glycerol 3-phosphate for gluconeogenesis.

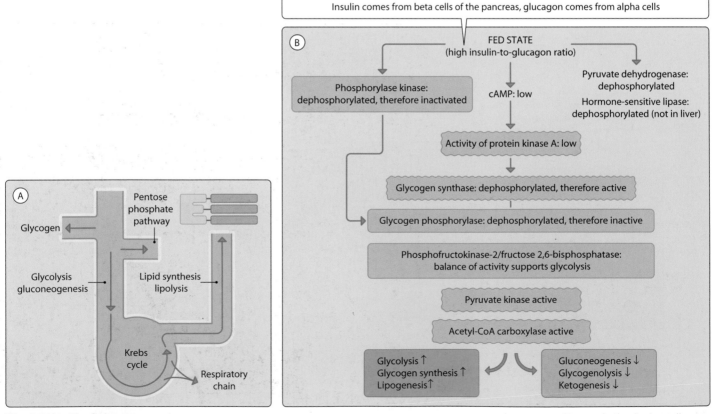

Fig. 3.51.1 The fed state.

About 80% of glucose uptake normally takes place in insulin-independent tissues (mainly the brain and the erythrocytes). In the fasting state, glucose uptake by insulin-dependent tissues reduces to spare glucose for these needs. After a 12 hours fast, up to 75% of circulating glucose is derived from the liver glycogen.

Gluconeogenesis successively increases during fasting. Low insulin concentration stimulates proteolysis and amino acids are released from muscle, mainly as alanine and glutamate, to serve as gluconeogenic substrates in the liver (this is known as the glucose–alanine cycle; Ch. 33). The increase in glucagon concentration stimulates lipolysis and fatty acid oxidation, which is a major source of acetyl-CoA. Depending on the availability of oxaloacetate, acetyl-CoA is channelled into either the Krebs cycle or ketogenesis. Fatty acids are the major fuel for muscle during prolonged exercise.

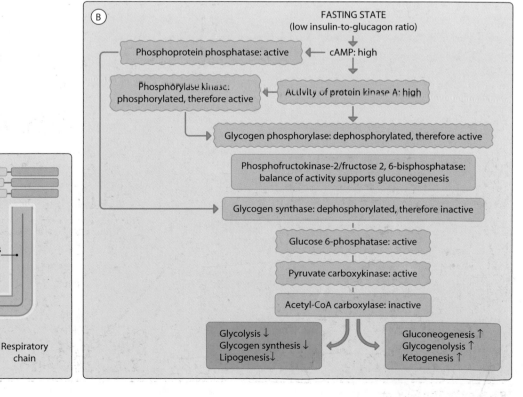

Fig. 3.51.2 The fasting state.

52. Insulin and glucagon I

Questions
- What is the role of insulin receptor substrate (IRS) in insulin action?
- What is insulin resistance?
- What is the metabolic syndrome?

Insulin

Structure and secretion

Insulin is secreted by the beta-cells in the pancreatic islets of Langerhans and is a two-chain polypeptide. Its A and B chains are linked by disulphide bridges. It is synthesized as a pro-hormone, preproinsulin, which is split to yield proinsulin. Proinsulin is proteolytically split further into insulin and the connecting peptide (C-peptide); both are secreted from the beta-cells in equimolar amounts. This is exploited by using C-peptide as a marker of residual insulin secretion in diabetic patients treated with insulin (this is mostly a research application).

Action

Insulin increases glucose uptake in muscle and adipose tissue. Most of the peripheral glucose uptake takes place in muscle (85%); adipose tissue accounts for only about 10% of the total uptake. In muscle and adipose tissue, insulin increases glucose transport, recruiting the glucose transporter GLUT4 to the membrane (Fig. 3.52.1). In the liver, glucose transport (but not intracellular glucose metabolism) is insulin independent.

Insulin signalling

Being a polypeptide hormone, insulin does not cross the cell membrane. Its action is mediated by a membrane receptor and downstream signalling cascades (Fig. 3.52.1 and Ch. 14). Insulin first binds to the α-subunit of its membrane receptor. This activates the β-subunit, which is a tyrosine kinase, leading to tyrosine autophosphorylation. The receptor also phosphorylates four proteins belonging to the insulin receptor substrate (IRS) family, and several others such as Shc, Gab-1 and Cbl. Phosphorylated IRS proteins interact with the regulatory subunit of phosphoinositide 3-kinase. This generates phosphoinositol phosphates, which, in turn, control serine/threonine protein kinases such as protein kinase B (Akt kinase). Phosphorylation of Shc and Gab-1 leads to activation of the mitogen-activated protein kinase (MAPK) pathway and, similarly to protein kinase B, contributes to the stimulation of glucose transport by increasing the translocation of the GLUT4 transporter from the cytoplasm to the plasma membrane.

> *Glucose transporters.* Note that there are several types of glucose transporter: GLUT2 is present in liver kidney and pancreatic beta-cells, GLUT4 occurs in muscle and adipose tissue, and GLUT5 in the intestine (p. 53).

Glucagon

Structure and secretion and action of glucagon

Glucagon is secreted by the alpha-cells in the pancreatic islets of Langerhans. It is a relatively small peptide with a molecular mass of 3485 Da.

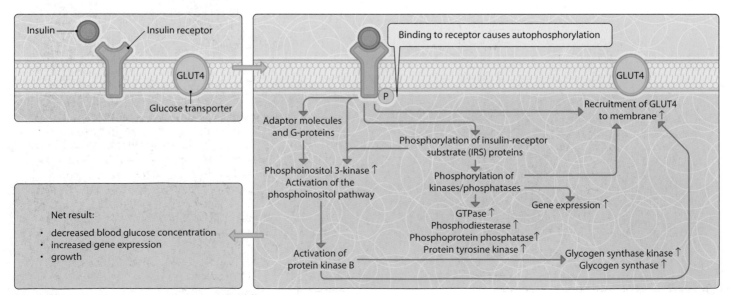

Fig. 3.52.1 The mechanism of action of insulin.

Action

Glucagon acts on the liver. It inhibits glucose utilization (glycolysis) and suppresses its storage (glycogen synthesis) while stimulating both glycogen breakdown (glucogenolysis) and glucose production from non-carbohydrate sources (gluconeogenesis). It also promotes lipolysis. All this is accomplished by phosphorylation of relevant enzymes and by repression and derepression of genes.

Glucagon signalling

The action of glucagon is a classic example of a hormone whose action is mediated by a G-protein–cAMP cascade (see Fig. 3.53.2 and Ch. 14).

Insulin resistance

Insulin resistance is a key factor associated with obesity and type 2 diabetes. It is defined as unresponsiveness of target tissues to insulin. It results in impaired cellular glucose uptake in adipose tissue and skeletal muscle (see Fig. 3.56.3). Insulin resistance is characterized by hyperinsulinaemia occurring together with glucose intolerance.

Insulin resistance, particularly in combination with defective insulin secretion, causes deterioration of glucose tolerance, leading first to impaired fasting glucose concentration (IFG), then to impaired glucose tolerance (IGT) and finally to overt diabetes mellitus. IFG and IGT are regarded as prediabetic conditions.

Insulin resistance is predominantly caused by defective insulin signalling (Fig. 3.52.2). In type 2 diabetes, the glucose transporter GLUT4 is downregulated, insulin binding to its receptor is reduced, receptor phosphorylation and tyrosine kinase activity are decreased, and there is decreased phosphorylation of insulin receptor substrate (IRS) proteins. This impairs insulin-stimulated glucose uptake in muscle. There is also increased synthesis and secretion of very low density lipoproteins by the liver.

The insulin resistance syndrome

Insulin resistance is associated with obesity (particularly central obesity: excessive fat tissue in and around the abdomen), and leads to glucose intolerance. It may occur in combination with other risk factors for cardiovascular disease, such as dyslipidaemia (mainly high triacylglycerols and low HDL-cholesterol) and hypertension, and also with low-grade inflammation and a state promoting thrombotic phenomena.

Importantly, the sequence obesity→metabolic-syndrome→type 2 diabetes mellitus may be prevented by lifestyle interventions such as weight reduction, diet and increased physical activity.

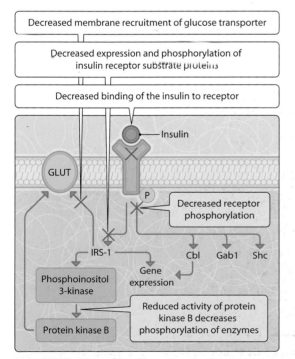

Fig. 3.52.2 Sites of insulin resistance (compare with Fig. 3.52.1).

 THE INSULIN RESISTANCE SYNDROME

A 32-year-old rugby player had to stop playing after injuring his knee. He then worked as a web designer. Two years later, he had gained 12 kg in weight; his blood pressure was 150/91 mmHg on two occasions (recommended value < 140/90 mmHg), and his plasma glucose was 6.5 mmol/l. He was prescribed hypotensive treatment and advised to loose weight and return to moderate regular exercise.

This man had developed the insulin resistance syndrome, the hallmarks of which are obesity, hypertension and glucose intolerance. Another frequent feature is dyslipidaemia, characterized by elevated triacylglycerol concentration and a low HDL-cholesterol, with total cholesterol remaining most of the time within the acceptable range.

53. Insulin and glucagon II: regulation of fuel metabolism

Questions
- How does insulin action result in the accumulation of body fat?
- What is the role of insulin receptor substrate (IRS)?
- Give an example of an enzyme that is reciprocally regulated by insulin and glucagon

The two pancreatic hormones, insulin and glucagon, are key controllers of metabolic fuel distribution during the fast–feed cycle. Normally, plasma glucose is kept within a narrow range (around 5 mmol/l, with increases after meals to less than 11 mmol/l). Insulin is an anabolic hormone that promotes glucose uptake into cells and the storage of fuels as triacylglycerols. It is the only hypoglycaemic hormone; its effects are countered by an array of hormones with hyperglycaemic action (the counter-regulatory hormones), the most important of which are glucagon, epinephrine and cortisol. Insulin and glucagon are peptides; epinephrine is an amino acid derivative and cortisol is a steroid. Insulin, glucagon and epinephrine have widespread effects on enzyme phosphorylation and, thus, modulation of enzyme activity (Fig. 3.53.1).

The metabolic cycle associated with fasting and feeding is controlled primarily by the ratio of concentrations of insulin and glucagon. Epinephrine and cortisol are particularly important in orchestrating body reaction to stress and trauma: epinephrine's action is instantaneous and cortisol is more important in chronic response to stress. Figure 3.53.2 summarizes the main metabolic effects of insulin and glucagon.

Note that glucagon and epinephrine are the main two hormones stimulating gluconeogenesis. Glycogenolysis in the liver is activated by both glucagon and epinephrine, but in muscle it is only epinephrine, acting through the β-adrenoceptor, that promotes glycogen degradation.

Insulin action
Insulin stimulates glycogen synthesis in the liver and muscle by activating glycogen synthase (Fig. 3.52.1). Insulin increases fatty acid and triacylglycerol synthesis in the liver by activating acetyl-CoA carboxylase (low insulin concentration reduces lipogenesis). It also increases the activity of lipoprotein lipase, promoting hydrolysis of triacylglycerols in very low density lipoproteins and chylomicrons. In the adipose tissue, insulin increases glucose uptake, conversion of glucose to fatty acids, and fatty acid esterification, and inhibits lipolysis.

Insulin suppresses gluconeogenesis. Ketogenesis is also suppressed at high insulin concentrations. Insulin promotes aerobic oxidation of glucose by activating pyruvate dehydrogenase. Finally, it increases protein synthesis and inhibits proteolysis.

Glucagon action
Glucagon binds to a membrane receptor. This binding causes GTP to bind to a G-protein complex, stimulating the dissociation of G-protein subunits, one of which stimulates adenylyl cyclase. This results in the production of cAMP and the activation of cAMP-dependent protein kinase A, which then phosphorylates key regulatory enzymes participating in glycolysis,

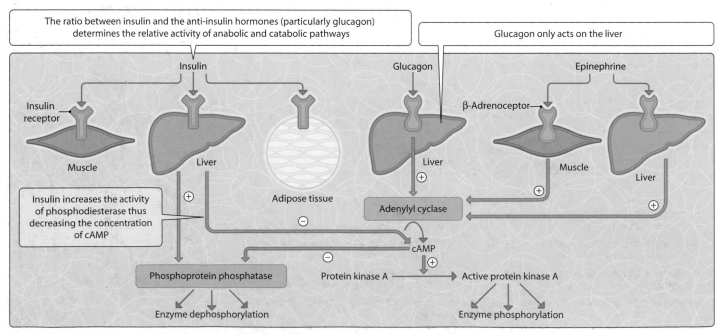

Fig. 3.53.1 The effect of insulin, glucagon and epinephrine on enzyme phosphorylation.

gluconeogenesis and lipolysis. (See Ch. 14 for examples of regulatory cascades.)

Hyperglycaemia and hypoglycaemia

The relative concentrations of insulin and the anti-insulin hormones affect the concentraton of plasma glucose. Figure 3.53.3 summarizes the main causes of hypo- and hyperglycaemia.

The oral glucose tolerance test

The normal response to a standard carbohydrate load is release of insulin and a rapid fall in plasma glucose concentration. This change in plasma glucose does not occur in diabetes mellitus. This oral glucose tolerance test has served for

decades as a test to diagnose diabetes mellitus in borderline cases. It is used less now as the fasting glucose concentration has similar diagnostic value. For the purposes of patient assessment, an overnight fast is regarded as the basal metabolic state. To obtain meaningful results from laboratory tests, it is important to measure substances that change during the fast–feed cycle such as glucose and triacylglycerols.

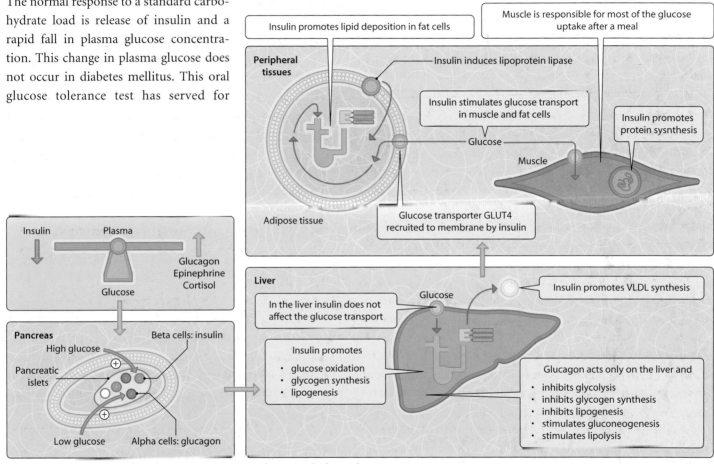

Fig. 3.53.2 The effect of insulin and glucagon on key metabolic pathways.

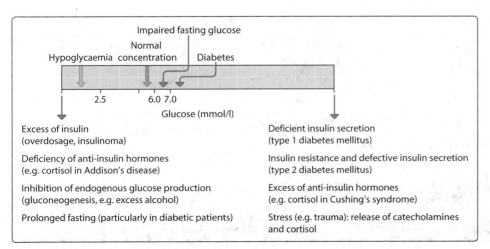

Fig. 3.53.3 Hypoglycaemia and hyperglycaemia.

HYPOGLYCAEMIA

Mild hypoglycaemia is the most common complication of insulin-dependent diabetes and may also occur in non-diabetic individuals. Symptoms of pallor sweating, tachycardia and hand tremor are resolved by an intake of sugar. Severe hypoglycaemia is a medical emergency and requires treatment with intravenous glucose infusion.

54. Metabolic aspects of exercise

Questions
- What is the role of troponins in muscle contraction?
- What is the role of intracellular calcium concentration in muscle contraction?
- What are the sources of muscle ATP during short- and long-term work?

Muscle

Muscle tissue is controlled by nerve impulses (both voluntary and involuntary).

In contractile cells, the cytoskeleton is modified to provide the contractile machinery. Shortening in muscle cells is mediated by the progressive overlap of interdigitated thick (myosin) and thin (F-actin) filaments. Myosin molecules contain two heavy and two light chains, which provide a head group for interaction with actin and a catalytic ATPase domain. Tropomyosin and troponin move in response to raised Ca^{2+} and allow activity of the contractile machinery. The opposite movement of thick and thin filaments during contraction is achieved by a cyclic interaction between attachment, pulling and detachment driven by the myosin head groups and the myosin ATPase activity.

In smooth and cardiac muscle, calcium ions interact with a binding protein **calmodulin** instead of with troponin C.

Metabolism during exercise

At rest, skeletal muscle is dependent on fatty acid oxidation. During short bursts of contraction, ATP required for contraction is instantly replenished from a high-energy compound, **creatine phosphate** (Fig. 3.54.1), in a reaction catalysed by **creatine kinase** and producing creatine and ATP. **Adenylate kinase** also replenishes ATP through the breakdown of ADP to AMP. AMP is subsequently deaminated to IMP, which stimulates glycogen phosphorylase and, thus, glycogen breakdown. Epinephrine also activates phosphorylase. In addition, the entry of calcium ions into the cytoplasm activates phosphofructokinase-1, stimulating glycolysis from the glycogen-derived glucose 6-phosphate.

Glycogen can support exercising muscle for about 1 hour (Fig. 3.54.2). However, as early as after 15–20 minutes of exercise, fatty acids, mobilized by the low insulin-to-glucagon ratio, become the principal fuel. Acetyl-CoA generated during fatty acid oxidation inhibits pyruvate dehydrogenase, conserving glycogen. Soon after, gluconeogenesis stimulated by epinephrine starts to produce de novo synthesized glucose. During recovery from exercise, lactate produced in anaerobic glycolysis is converted into glucose (the glucose–lactate cycle; Fig. 3.32.2).

Interrelations between carbohydrate and fat metabolism
Continuing supply of glucose (by glycolysis or by ingestion) is important to maintain efficient fat oxidation. Pyruvate provided by glycolysis replenishes oxaloacetate, depleted by gluconeogenesis, in an anaplerotic reaction catalysed by pyruvate carboxylase (see Ch. 38). Other anaplerotic reactions supply oxaloacetate through succinyl-CoA production from the amino acids valine and isoleucine.

The insulin-like effect of exercise
Exercise increases glucose uptake by increasing the recruitment of GLUT4 to the cell membrane; this effect is similar to the action of insulin. Because of this insulin-like effect, diabetic persons need to reduce their insulin dose before intense exercise.

Energy expenditure during physical activity
A conventional way presenting energy expenditure associated with exercise is to do so in multiples of the basal metabolic rate. Table 3.54.1 presents the energy expenditure associated with common activities.

Markers of muscle damage
Destruction of myocytes is associated with release of enzymes and proteins from the sarcoplasm. These (myoglobin and creatine kinase) are used in the diagnosis of skeletal muscle disorders and, in particular, in the diagnosis of myocardial infarction (ischaemia-induced necrosis of the cardiac muscle). As creatine kinase occurs as different isozymes in different tissues, the origin of raised plasma creatine kinase can be determined. The MB

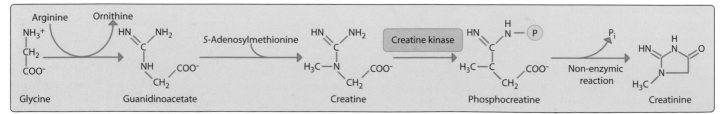

Fig. 3.54.1 Creatine, creatine kinase and creatine phosphate.

Table 3.54.1 ENERGY EXPENDITURE DURING PHYSICAL ACTIVITY

Activity level	Energy requirement related to BMR (mets)[a]	Energy usage (kJ/min (kcal/min))	Description
Light	< 3	< 17 (< 4)	Slow walking (1–2 mph), slow swimming, using a vacuum cleaner, weeding the garden
Moderate	3–6	17–29 (4–7)	Brisk walking (3–4 mph), cycling (5–10 mph), swimming with moderate exertion, heavier home cleaning, mowing grass with a power mower
Vigerous	> 6	> 29 (> 7)	Walking uphill briskly, cycling (> 10 mph), swimming fast, moving furniture, digging garden

[a]Metabolic equivalents (mets) are the energy requirement expressed as a multiple of the energy requirement at rest (the basal metabolic rate (BMR)).

isoenzyme of CK (CK-MB) has been used for a long time as a cardiac marker in the diagnosis of myocardial infarction. This has now been substituted by the measurements of cardiac troponins. Figure 3.54.3 shows the most important cardiac markers and the timescale of their release after the myocardial infarction.

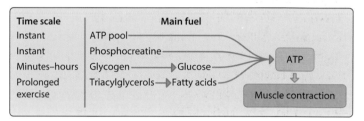

Fig. 3.54.2 Metabolic fuels used during exercise.

 MYOCARDIAL INFARCTION

Heart attack
A 70-year-old woman felt chest discomfort which she thought was indigestion after a large breakfast. However, after about 20 minutes, the pain become crushing in nature. She was rushed to a hospital where a myocardial infarction was diagnosed on the basis of her symptoms and the electrocardiograph. There were no contraindications to thrombolytic treatment and she was immediately given streptokinase. Her plasma cardiac troponin concentration was grossly elevated.

Silent myocardial infarction
A fit 52-year-old former long-distance runner had been feeling sufficiently unwell that he stopped his habitual 5 mile run for a few days. Ten days later he attended a specialist clinic to have a routine check of his cholesterol level. A routine electrocardiograph demonstrated an old inferior myocardial infarction. This was confirmed by the echocardiogram, which showed impaired inferior wall motility. This man had had a so-called silent myocardial infarction. He was subsequently treated with aspirin and a beta blocker, in addition to lipid-lowering therapy.

The measurements of cardiac troponins (troponin C or troponin I) are the main laboratory tests in the diagnosis of myocardial infarction

Troponin	——
Myoglobin	——
CK-MB	——
Total creatine kinase (CK)	——

Time (days)

The MB isoform of CK is specific for heart

Fig. 3.54.3 The markers of cardiac muscle injury.

55. Metabolic aspects of stress and injury

Questions
- What is the role of epinephrine in stress response?
- Why should glucose intolerance not be diagnosed during an acute illness?
- What is the commonly used laboratory marker of infection?

Stress, trauma and injury induce a catabolic state.

The response to trauma, infection and stress is directed by the central nervous system (CNS) (Fig. 3.55.1). The emotional and physical stimuli are integrated in the hypothalamus, which secretes corticotrophin-releasing hormone (CRH), stimulating the pituitary. The pituitary responds with the secretion of adrenocorticotrophic hormone (ACTH), which, in turn, stimulates cortisol production in the adrenal cortex.

In parallel, the stimulation of the sympathetic nervous system leads to increased catecholamine release from the adrenal medulla. The combined effects of catecholamines and cortisol retune energy metabolism towards the supply of glucose for the 'fight and flight' reaction.

Metabolic changes in stress
Stress, trauma and injury are associated with increased O_2 consumption.

Epinephrine, acting through adrenoceptors and the G-protein–adenylyl cyclase cascade, induces the anti-insulin response: primarily glycogenolysis and gluconeogenesis (Fig. 3.55.2). Lack of insulin leads to decreased peripheral glucose uptake, thus conserving glucose for the brain and the erythrocytes. In chronic stress, lipolysis and fatty acid oxidation are stimulated in parallel with gluconeogenesis. Muscle proteolysis increases. Cortisol plays a permissive role in the stimulation of gluconeogenesis by catecholamines and glucagon.

Plasma glucose concentration during stress
The response to stress and injury is characterized by mild hyperglycaemia. However, diabetes mellitus, if present, may become decompensated. Indeed, it is not uncommon that diabetes is diagnosed after illness or injury.

Stress and protein synthesis: the acute phase response
The so-called acute phase response is a major change in protein synthesis pattern, particularly in the liver, observed during illness or injury. There is an increase in the synthesis of α_1-antitrypsin, fibrinogen and C-reactive protein (CRP), and suppression of albumin synthesis. Measurement of CRP is commonly used as a marker of ongoing infection.

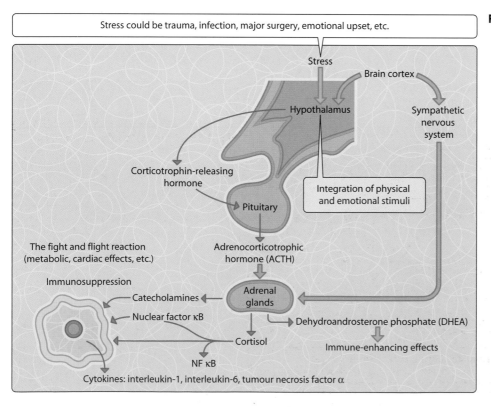

Fig. 3.55.1 The pathways in stress.

Stress could be trauma, infection, major surgery, emotional upset, etc.

Stress

Brain cortex

Hypothalamus

Sympathetic nervous system

Corticotrophin-releasing hormone

Integration of physical and emotional stimuli

Pituitary

The fight and flight reaction (metabolic, cardiac effects, etc.)

Adrenocorticotrophic hormone (ACTH)

Immunosuppression

Catecholamines

Adrenal glands

Nuclear factor κB

Dehydroandrosterone phosphate (DHEA)

Cortisol

Immune-enhancing effects

NF κB

Cytokines: interleukin-1, interleukin-6, tumour necrosis factor α

Stress and the immune system

The 'fight and flight' response is associated with suppression of the immune system. The inflammatory response is mediated by cytokines, particularly tumour necrosis factor-α, interleukin-1 and interleukin-6, which are secreted by resident tissue macrophages. Cortisol decreases the production of these pro-inflammatory cytokines. The glucocorticoid receptor reverses the activation of NFκB, a transcription factor that mediates the inflammatory response.

However, other hormones such as the adrenal steroid dehydroepiandrosterone (DHEA) may balance this immunosuppression by stimulating different parts of the inflammatory response (Fig. 3.55.1). The balance between immunosuppressant and immunostimulatory aspects of the stress response is fundamental for clinical outcome. Infections and generalized conditions associated with suppressed immunity, such as the adult respiratory distress syndrome (ARDS) and multiple organ failure, remain major concerns in patients who sustain trauma. These considerations also apply to major surgical procedures.

INTERPRETATION OF LABORATORY TESTS

A 50-year-old lady was admitted to the hospital with worsening breathlessness. She had been a heavy smoker for many years and had a history of congestive obstructive pulmonary disease and emphysema. Pneumonia was diagnosed on the basis of radiographic findings and *Staphylococcus aureus* was grown from the sputum culture. Her temperature was 39°C and the CRP concentration was 250 mg/l. On routine investigations, her fasting plasma glucose was 7.5 mmol/l (7 mmol/l is the diagnostic cut-off point for diabetes mellitus).

Diabetes was not diagnosed at that point, but an appointment was arranged with the GP to repeat the glucose measurement 6 weeks after her return home. This is because the stress response associated with a severe infection leads to the release of anti-insulin hormones and increased endogenous glucose production and elevated plasma glucose. Diabetes should not be diagnosed at this time if borderline values are observed. (Note, however, that ketoacidosis might be precipitated by infection or trauma in a previously undiagnosed diabetic person.)

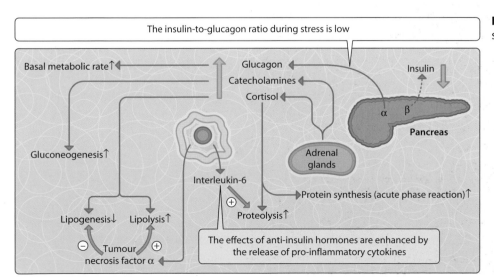

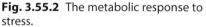

Fig. 3.55.2 The metabolic response to stress.

56. Obesity

Questions
- Give examples of adipokines. How can they contribute to insulin resistance?
- What pathological conditions are linked to obesity?
- What is the metabolic syndrome?

Obesity has increased worldwide by more than 70% since 1980. It is a major risk factor for type 2 diabetes mellitus. Similar to type 2 diabetes, obesity is characterized by insulin resistance. Obesity is classified with reference to the **body mass index** (BMI):

- 25–29.9: overweight
- 30–39.9: obesity
- 40+: gross obesity.

Adipose tissue is an active endocrine organ

Adipose tissue is an active endocrine organ. Its secretory products, **adipokines**, include:

- **adiponectin**, which enhances insulin sensitivity: in the liver adiponectin decreases gluconeogenesis and in muscle it increases the membrane transport of fatty acids
- **leptin**, which decreases appetite and increases thermogenesis: its concentration in plasma is proportional to body fat content and it may promote lipid oxidation and inhibit lipid synthesis in muscle
- **resistin**, which induces severe insulin resistance in animals
- **growth factors** such as vascular endothelial growth factor
- **pro-inflammatory cytokines** such as tumour necrosis factor-α and interleukin-6 (the former decreases the expression of the muscle glucose transporter GLUT4).

Control of food intake

Food intake is controlled by hunger (a desire to eat) and appetite (a desire for a particular food) (Fig. 3.56.1). Signals that control food intake originate in the adipose tissue and are processed by the central nervous system (CNS) (Fig. 3.56.2). The brain then

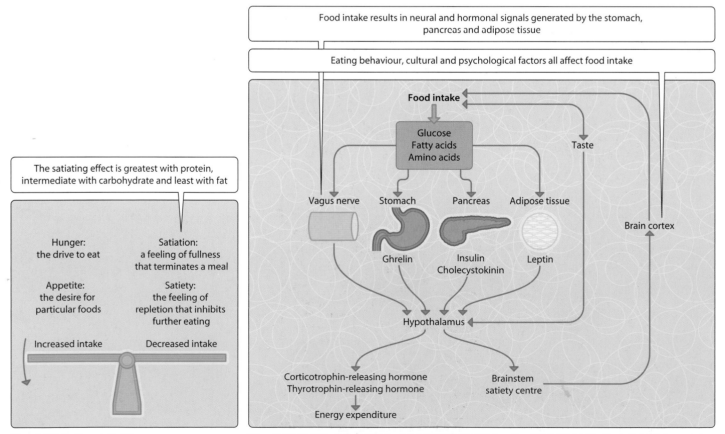

Fig. 3.56.1 Key definitions.

Fig. 3.56.2 The integration of cortical, hypothalamic and metabolic signals in the regulations of food intake.

generates neuropeptides that regulate appetite and hunger. Insulin and leptin act on the central neurons in the brain that control appetite and energy expenditure. These signals are conveyed by two neuropeptides: catabolic **proopiomelatocortin (POMC)**, and anabolic **neuropeptide Y/agouti-related protein (NPY/AgRP)**. POMC gives rise to melanocortins, which decrease food intake. NPY/AgRP links to neurons that connect with the brain's 'satiety centre' to promote hunger and to stimulate yet another set of hormones, such as corticotrophin-releasing hormone (CRH), thyrotrophin-releasing hormone (TRH), that increase thermogenesis and food intake. Other signals involved in the control of food intake are mediated by gastrointestinal peptides such as glucagon, cholecystokinin, glucagon-like peptide, amylin and bombesin-like peptide. **Ghrelin**, secreted by the stomach, is the only known appetite-stimulating peptide.

Obesity, insulin resistance and diabetes

Obesity is associated with insulin resistance and the metabolic syndrome (Ch. 52). Both are associated with dyslipidaemia, although not with the type characterized by high concentrations of low density lipoprotein (LDL)-cholesterol. The metabolic flux in obesity is illustrated in Fig. 3.44.3. Obesity increases the risk of developing arterial hypertension and is associated with cardiovascular disease. Associations observed between obesity, diabetes and cardiovascular disease led to the development of the 'common soil' hypothesis and the concept of diabesity, obesity-associated diabetes. It seems that the low-grade inflammatory reaction seen in particular in the arterial walls could be a common denominator between these conditions (Fig. 3.56.3).

WEIGHT REDUCTION

To lose weight one needs to change the balance between energy intake and expenditure: food intake needs to balance with energy expenditure in routine body activities and physical activity to give efficiency of use versus strage of energy. Low-calorie diets contain approximately 1200–1300 kcal/day and the very-low-calorie diets contain approximately 800 kcal/day. Generally a combination of diet and exercise is more effective in inducing weight loss than diet alone. A low-carbohydrate, high-fat diet appears to be effective in weight reduction.

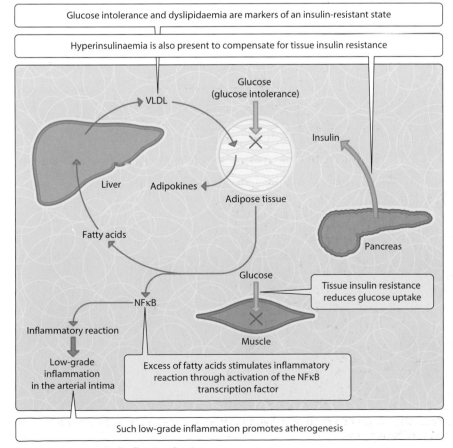

Fig. 3.56.3 Metabolic flux in obesity.

57. Diabetes mellitus

Questions
- Compare and contrast type 1 and type 2 diabetes
- How does diabetic ketoacidosis develop?
- What are the principles of treatment of hypoglycaemia?

Diabetes mellitus is characterized by hyperglycaemia and by the risk, of long-term vascular complications (Fig. 3.57.1). It is caused by

- insulin deficiency, precipitated by the autoimmune destruction of the pancreatic islets (type 1 diabetes)
- a parallel decline in insulin secretion and increase in tissue insulin resistance (type 2 diabetes).

The diagnostic criteria are identical for both types (Table 3.57.1). Clinical symptoms are also similar. There are some differences in long-term complications: while microangiopathy is more pronounced in type 1 diabetes, cardiovascular disease features more prominently in type 2.

Type 1 and type 2 diabetes constitute the so-called primary diabetes mellitus (approximately 90% of all diabetic patients have type 2 diabetes). Secondary diabetes may develop in conditions of excess of anti-insulin hormones such as cortisol (Cushing syndrome) or growth hormone, or when pancreatic islets are destroyed by pancreatitis. In haemochromatosis, a disorder of iron metabolism, pancreatic fibrosis may also lead to diabetes.

During the development of diabetes mellitus there is a continuity between glucose intolerance and overt diabetes mellitus. Obesity is a major risk factor for both. In some patients, the transition from glucose intolerance to diabetes can be prevented or delayed by lifestyle changes such as weight reduction and increased exercise.

The effects of insulin lack

The metabolic flux in diabetes is illustrated in Figure 3.57.2. Lack of insulin produces potentially life-threatening metabolic changes (Fig. 3.57.3). The net effect is the predominance of the effect of glucagon and hyperglycaemic hormones. This leads to:

- decreased peripheral glucose uptake and increased hepatic production of glucose, resulting in hyperglycaemia
- increased lipolysis, which generates excess acetyl-CoA and stimulates ketogenesis.

Osmotic effects of glucose in diabetes

When plasma glucose concentration reaches approximately 10 mmol/l, the renal transport system in the proximal tubule becomes overwhelmed and glucose enters urine. During its journey through the renal tubule, glucose osmotically attracts water; consequently, the volume of urine and the frequency of urination increases (**polyuria**). This is called **osmotic diuresis**. Not treated, it results in dehydration.

Diabetic ketoacidosis

Accumulation of acidic ketone bodies leads to diabetic ketoacidosis. The three hallmarks of decompensated type 1 diabetes are acidosis, dehydration and hyperglycaemia. Diabetic ketoacidosis is a medical emergency.

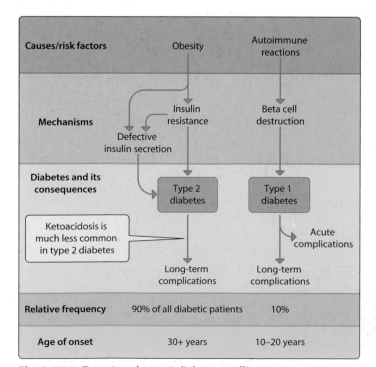

Fig. 3.57.1 Type 1 and type 2 diabetes mellitus.

Table 3.57.1 DIAGNOSTIC CRITERIA FOR GLUCOSE INTOLERANCE AND DIABETES MELLITUS

Status	Fasting glucose (mmol/l (mg/dl))	2 h after a 75 g glucose load (mmol/l (mg/dl))
Normal	< 6.1 (< 110)	–
Impaired fasting glucose (IFG)	6.1–7.0 (110–126)	–
Impaired glucose tolerance (IGT)	–	7.8-11.1 (140–200)
Diabetes mellitus	> 7 (> 126)	> 11.1 (> 200)

The sequence of events leading to diabetic ketoacidosis is illustrated in Figure 3.57.3. Clinically, diabetic ketoacidosis is characterized by dehydration and fast shallow breathing (Kussmaul breathing), resulting from the respiratory compensation of metabolic acidosis. There is high blood glucose, ketones in blood and glucose and ketones in urine.

Treatment of diabetic ketoacidosis

Treatment of ketoacidosis consists of rehydration and insulin infusion. Only in extreme cases is the correction of acidosis required.

Hypoglycaemia

Hypoglycaemia is blood glucose concentration < 2.5 mmol/l. It may be life threatening because normally glucose is the only fuel the brain can use. In general, hypoglycaemia occurs when the effects of insulin prevail over those of anti-insulin hormones. Hypoglycaemia may be caused by many different factors (see also Ch. 53).

In insulin-treated patients, hypoglycaemia is most often caused by a missed meal or inadvertent increase in insulin dose. Exercise has an insulin-like effect and the dose of insulin needs to be decreased before intense exercise. Alcohol causes hypoglycaemia through the inhibition of gluconeogenesis.

The majority of hypoglycaemic episodes are mild and many healthy people experience hypoglycaemia at some point after, for instance, intensive exercise during fasting. Severe hypoglycaemia, however, is a medical emergency.

TYPE 2 DIABETES

A 58-year-old woman gained 11 kg in weight over 3 years and her BMI reached 32. She complained of extreme tiredness and needed to get up several times a night to pass urine. She drank 2–3 litres of fluid a day. Her mother and a maternal aunt were both known to have diabetes. She had fasting glucose 13.5 mmol/l (reference range < 7 mmol/l); glucosuria but no ketones in urine.

This woman had developed type 2 diabetes, which is clearly linked to obesity. The symptoms of developing diabetes may be non-specific but polyuria and polydypsia are important pointers.

DIABETIC KETOACIDOSIS

A 13-year-old previously healthy girl became acutely ill after a few days of a 'flu-like illness. She became drowsy, confused, appeared dehydrated and her breath smelled of acetone. Her blood glucose concentration was 27 mmol/l and there were large amounts of ketones in her urine. Diabetic ketoacidosis was diagnosed and she was treated with intravenous fluids and the infusion of short-acting insulin.

Diabetic ketoacidosis may be precipitated by other illness and, as in this case, may be the first presentation of type 1 diabetes.

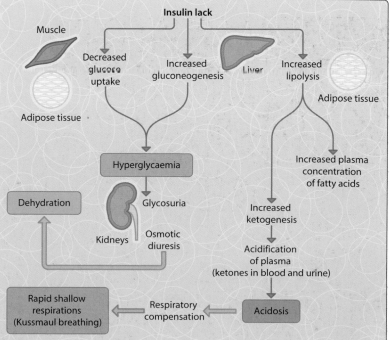

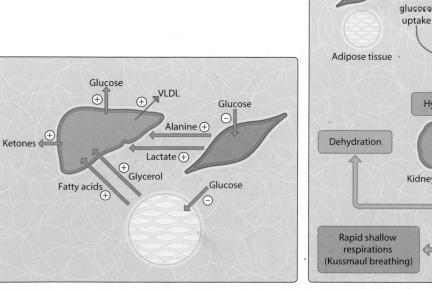

Fig. 3.57.2 Metabolism in diabetes mellitus.

Fig. 3.57.3 The effects of insulin lack and the development of diabetes ketoacidosis.

58. Long-term complications of diabetes mellitus

Questions
- How would you diagnose diabetic nephropathy?
- What are the most important tests used to monitor glycaemic control?
- What is the relationship between glycated haemoglobin and the advanced glycosylation end-products?

Long-term complications of diabetes (Fig. 3.58.1) include:

- diabetic eye disease (retinopathy)
- kidney disease (nephropathy)
- peripheral nerve disease (neuropathy).

Diabetes is also strongly associated with atherosclerosis. Retinopathy and nephropathy affect small arteries and are known as **diabetic microangiopathy**. Atherosclerosis affects large vessels and in this setting is known as **macroangiopathy**.

Development of long-term complications

Long-term complications result from the toxicity of glucose and fatty acids and the damage inflicted by reactive oxygen species (ROS) (Fig. 3.58.2).

Glucotoxicity and lipotoxicity

It has been known for a long time that glucose is a reducing agent: it can become oxidized when reacting with metals such as copper. This yields superoxide and hydrogen peroxide. Glucose can also react with proteins in a process known as **glycation** (Fig. 3.58.3). Glycation and oxidation form a common path, and the entire process became known as **glycoxidation**. Autooxidation of glycated protein-bound residues (called Amadori products) yields superoxide and hydroxyl radicals as well as another group of reactive molecules, dicarbonyls. The result of glycoxidation is the formation of advanced glycation end-products (AGE),

Fig. 3.58.1 Long-term complications of diabetes mellitus.

Fig. 3.58.1 Long-term complications of diabetes mellitus.

Fig. 3.58.2 Diabetes and oxidant stress.

Fig. 3.58.3 Role of advanced glycation end-products in the development of the diabetic complications.

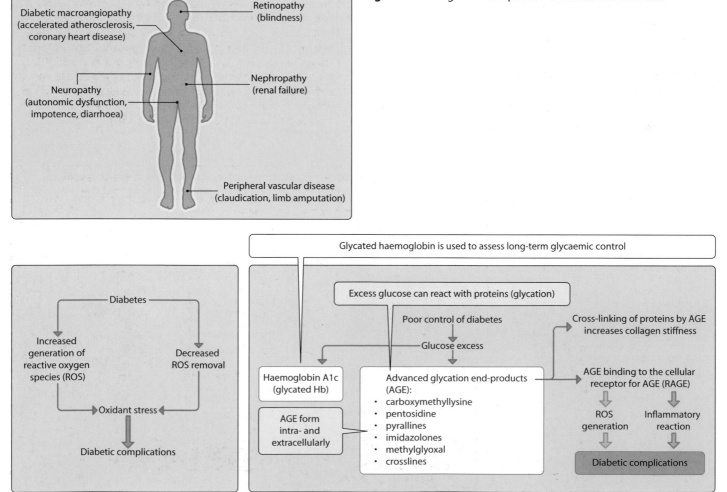

which form both extracellularly and intracellularly and serve as protein crosslinks. Such crosslinks are found, for example, on collagen in diabetes, making it 'stiffer' and less amenable to proteolytic degradation. Intracellular oxidation of glucose also yields glyoxal, methylglyoxal and 3-deoxyglucosone, which are reactive dicarbonyl compounds that react with the amino groups. AGE also bind to a membrane receptor (receptor for AGE: RAGE), which stimulates both inflammatory reactions and ROS generation (Fig. 3.58.3). Finally a polyol pathway (Fig. 3.58.4) may contribute to diabetic complications by generation of osmotically active sorbitol (thought important in the development of diabetic cataracts) and also by generation of AGE.

Oxidative stress

The plausible sequence of events leading to tissue damage caused by oxidative reactions is as follows. The mitochondrial respiratory chain normally produces ROS and this oxidative stress activates a protein kinase, protein kinase C. The abundance of glucose increases mitochondrial oxidations, leading to an increase in the proton gradient and concomitantly to increased mitochondrial ROS production. In addition to the excess ROS production, diabetes is characterized by reduced levels of glutathione and other antioxidant compounds. This contributes to the oxidative stress (Fig. 3.58.5).

Assessing long-term glycaemic control: haemoglobin A1c

Haemoglobin A1c (HbA1c) is a glycated form of haemoglobin A and is used as a marker of long-term glycaemic control.

Haemoglobin is non-enzymatically glycated at a rate proportional to the ambient glucose concentration. The glycation reaction is practically irreversible and the modified haemoglobin stays in the circulation for the entire life of an erythrocyte. This means that, at any time, its concentration reflects the average past glycaemia over a period of 4–6 weeks. The concentration of HbA1c is related to the frequency of diabetic complications. Measurement of HbA1c is a key index of glycaemic control used during the clinical assessment of diabetic patients.

MONITORING DIABETIC CONTROL

Monitoring diabetic (glycaemic) control is a key issue in diabetes care, because clinical studies such as the Diabetes Control and Complications Trial (DCCT; involving type 1 diabetic patients) and the UK Prospective Diabetes Study (UK PDS; involving type 2 diabetic patients) have demonstrated that maintaining near-normal plasma glucose concentration in diabetes decreases the incidence, and the rate of progression, of long-term complications.

Monitoring of diabetic patients involves a number of laboratory tests including regular testing of blood glucose, measurement of HbA1c and measurement of albumin excretion in urine. Albumin is measured with a sensitive method able to detect so-called microalbuminuria (i.e. microgram amounts of albumin), which indicate early stages of diabetic nephropathy. Monitoring of diabetic patients also includes measuring lipids—cholesterol, triacylglycerols and HDL-cholesterol—to detect dyslipidaemia and to assess the risk of cardiovascular disease. Diabetic patients need to have regular ophthalmic examinations to detect the presence of diabetic retinopathy (indicated by cotton-wool spots).

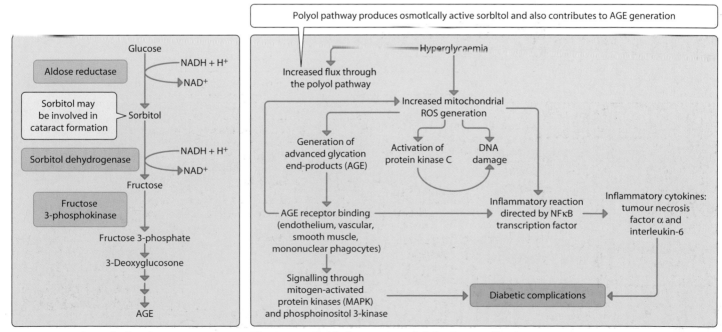

Fig. 3.58.4 The polyol pathway.

Fig. 3.58.5 Oxidative stress and diabetic complications.

59. Metabolic aspects of starvation and malnutrition

Questions
- What characterizes complicated malnutrition?
- How would one avoid the development of the refeeding syndrome?
- What is the metabolism of carbohydrates in prolonged fasting?

Malnutrition is a major problem in the developing world; in developed countries it can be seen during illness and hospital stay. Assessment of nutritional status should be an integral part of clinical examination.

Metabolic changes in starvation

During prolonged fasting, the insulin-to-glucagon ratio remains low and thyroid hormones also decrease. During fasting, the source of glucose changes from diet and glycogen to gluconeogenesis (Fig. 3.59.1) As fasting progresses, glucagon-stimulated lipolysis and fatty acid oxidation start to contribute. Gluconeogenesis exhausts the supply of oxaloacetate and acetyl-CoA is directed into ketogenesis. Ketone bodies become a fuel for muscle and, with time, the brain. The need for gluconeogenic substrates leads to the utilization of body protein as fuel. In this state, giving glucose to a starved person saves body protein by suppressing gluconeogenesis. In starvation the basal metabolic rate decreases (Fig. 3.59.2).

Malnutrition and nutritional deficiencies

Malnutrition, if advanced, leads to medical complications. Protein–energy malnutrition (PEM) is poor nutritional status owing to inadequate nutrient intake. In addition to protein and energy deficiency, specific deficiencies such as the iron deficiency, leading to anaemia, or those of vitamin D and vitamin C may develop. Two types of PEM may be observed in children: **marasmus** and **kwashiorkor** (Fig. 3.59.3).

Marasmus results from chronic inadequate intake of calories and protein, and it develops over months or years. There is loss of weight, muscle tissue and subcutaneous fat; synthesis of visceral proteins such as albumin is preserved.

Kwashiorkor is a more acute form of undernutrition, which may occur on the background of marasmus. It may also develop because of inadequate nutrient intake after trauma or infection. In contrast to marasmus, visceral tissues are not spared and there is oedema resulting from low plasma levels of albumin, which may mask weight loss. Complications of kwashiorkor are dehydration, hypoglycaemia, hypothermia and electrolyte disturbances. There is impaired immunity and wound healing and increased risk of infection. Recently, a proposed classification divides malnutrition into moderate, severe and complicated (Table 3.59.1).

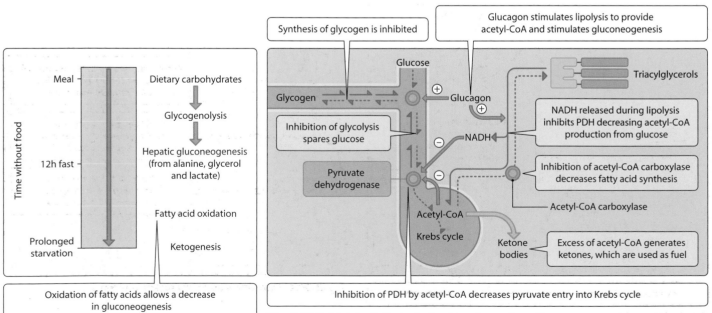

Fig. 3.59.1 Utilization of metabolic fuels during fasting and starvation.

Fig. 3.59.2 Metabolic fuels during long-term starvation.

Nutritional assessment

Assessment of nutritional status is an important part of general clinical examination both in hospital and in outpatient clinics.

The refeeding syndrome

A starved person needs to be repleted nutritionally slowly. Too quick a replacement is dangerous because it may cause major fluid shifts between intracellular and extracellular fluid. This is known as the refeeding syndrome and is characterized by low serum magnesium, phosphate and potassium ions. If thiamine deficiency is present, carbohydrate feeding can precipitate the Wernicke–Korsakoff syndrome. Therefore, in situations such as during famine relief, frequent simple meals at short intervals are recommended.

Table 3.59.1 CLASSIFICATION OF MALNUTRITION

Level of malnutrition	Median weight for height (%)	Characteristics
Moderate	70–80	No oedema, clinical well-being and alertness, the presence of appetite
Severe	< 70	Weight loss or the development of oedema
Complicated	< 80	Or oedema with a concomitant anorexia, respiratory infection, fever, dehydration or severe anaemia

From Collins S, Yates R 2003 The need to update the classification of acute malnutrition. Lancet 362: 249

 REFEEDING SYNDROME

A 26-year-old malnourished man developed sepsis after cholecystectomy. Standard intravenous nutrition regimen was commenced but within 2 days, he developed severe hypokalaemia, hypophosphataemia and hypomagnesaemia.

This patient, fed intensively after a prolonged period of fasting, showed major electrolyte disturbances: the biochemical signs of the refeeding syndrome. Gradual introduction of food with careful monitoring is essential to avoid this complication both in hospital and in famine areas.

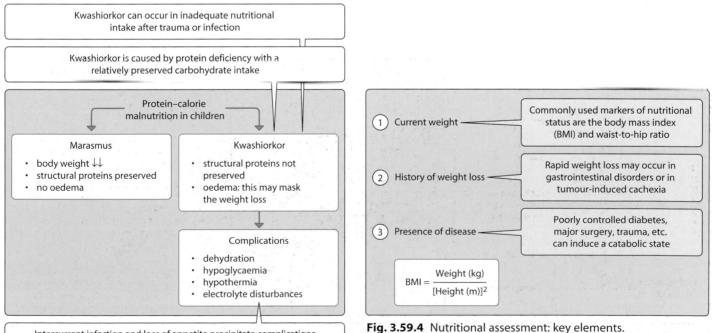

Fig. 3.59.3 Malnutrition.

Fig. 3.59.4 Nutritional assessment: key elements.

60. Atherosclerosis

Questions
- How do foam cells develop?
- What is the role of oxidative processes in the development of the atherosclerotic plaque?
- What are the main cardiovascular risk factors?

Atherosclerosis is a disease of the large arteries. It leads to functional impairment of vessel structure (remodelling) and function, together with formation of atherosclerotic plaque. The three major types of atherosclerotic disease (Fig. 3.60.1) are coronary heart disease, stroke and peripheral vascular disease. Cardiovascular disease is presently the leading cause of death

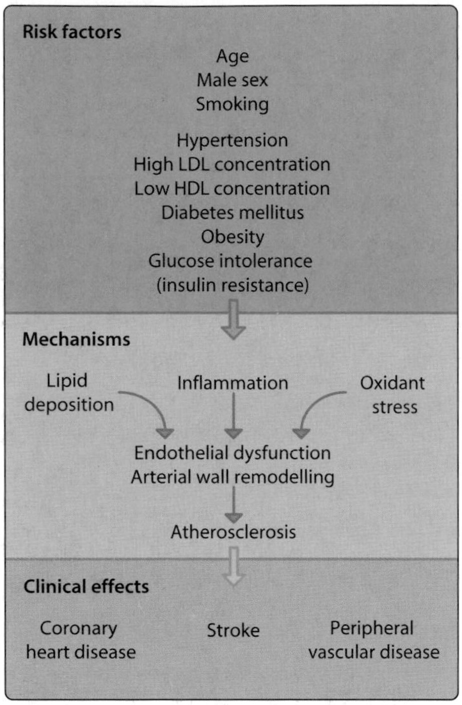

Fig. 3.60.1 Causes, risk factors for and clinical effects of atherosclerosis.

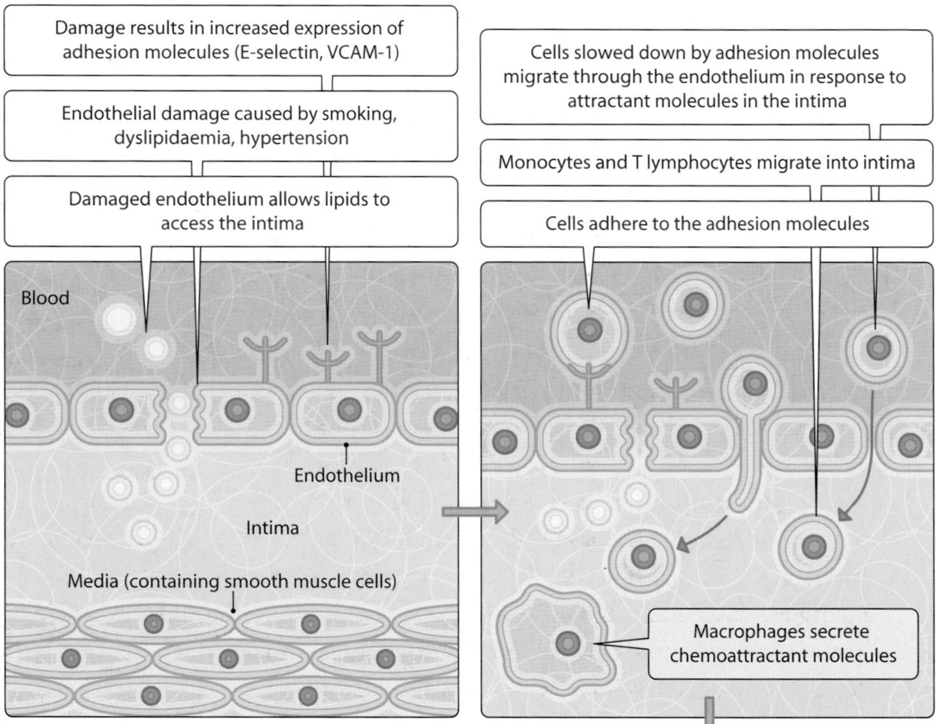

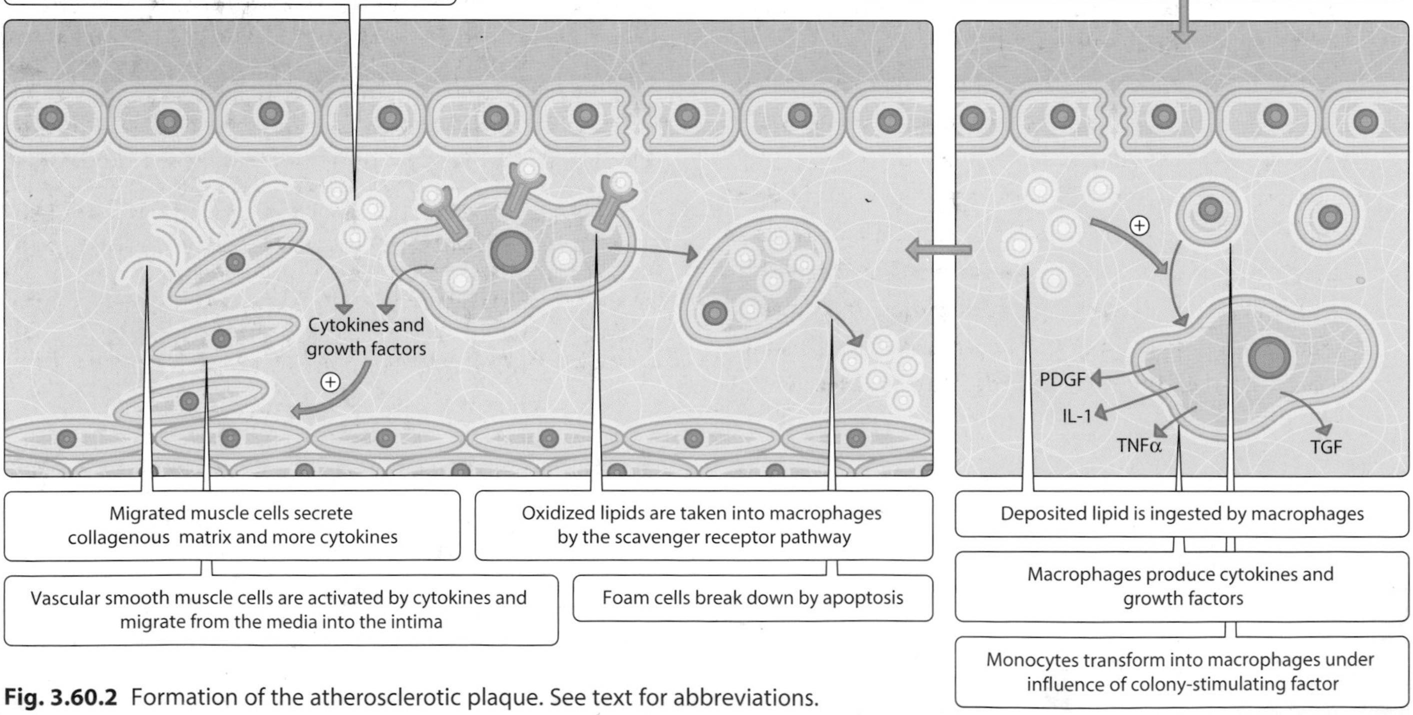

Risk factors
Age
Male sex
Smoking

Hypertension
High LDL concentration
Low HDL concentration
Diabetes mellitus
Obesity
Glucose intolerance
(insulin resistance)

Mechanisms
Lipid deposition   Inflammation   Oxidant stress

Endothelial dysfunction
Arterial wall remodelling

Atherosclerosis

Clinical effects
Coronary heart disease   Stroke   Peripheral vascular disease

Damage results in increased expression of adhesion molecules (E-selectin, VCAM-1)

Endothelial damage caused by smoking, dyslipidaemia, hypertension

Damaged endothelium allows lipids to access the intima

Blood

Endothelium

Intima

Media (containing smooth muscle cells)

Cells slowed down by adhesion molecules migrate through the endothelium in response to attractant molecules in the intima

Monocytes and T lymphocytes migrate into intima

Cells adhere to the adhesion molecules

Macrophages secrete chemoattractant molecules

Lipid oxidation takes place in the intima

Cytokines and growth factors

Migrated muscle cells secrete collagenous matrix and more cytokines

Vascular smooth muscle cells are activated by cytokines and migrate from the media into the intima

Oxidized lipids are taken into macrophages by the scavenger receptor pathway

Foam cells break down by apoptosis

PDGF
IL-1
TNFα   TGF

Deposited lipid is ingested by macrophages

Macrophages produce cytokines and growth factors

Monocytes transform into macrophages under influence of colony-stimulating factor

Fig. 3.60.2 Formation of the atherosclerotic plaque. See text for abbreviations.

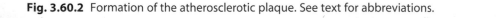

worldwide. However, it is not the chronic narrowing of the vessel that is the direct cause of acute ischaemic events such as myocardial infarction or stroke. It is the rupture of the atherosclerotic plaque that leads to thrombus formation and blockage of vascular lumen.

Formation of the atherosclerotic plaque

The atherosclerotic plaque is a result of several processes.

Endothelial damage. Atherosclerosis is initiated by functional impairment of the vascular endothelium (Fig. 3.60.2). Healthy endothelium has a smooth surface with antithrombotic and antiadhesive properties. Damaged endothelium expresses adhesion molecules such as vascular cell adhesion molecule-1 (VCAM-1) and monocyte chemotactic protein-1 (MCP-1); white blood cells such as monocytes can adhere to the vascular wall and migrate to the vascular intima. There, under the influence of the monocyte-colony-stimulating factor (M-CSF), they transform into resident macrophages.

Arterial deposition of lipoproteins. Lipoproteins (remnant particles and low density lipoproteins (LDL); see Ch. 22) penetrate the arterial wall and deposit in the intima. When they leave the circulation, they become more prone to oxidation by oxygen free radicals. Oxidized lipoproteins stimulate inflammatory reaction in the arterial wall and are taken up by macrophages, which become overloaded with lipids and transform into so-called **foam cells**. These cells eventually disintegrate, releasing lipid, which becomes a core of the forming atherosclerotic plaque.

Activation of arterial smooth muscle cells. Damaged endothelial cells secrete cytokines such as platelet-derived growth factor (PDGF), interleukin-1 (IL-1) and tumour necrosis factor (TNF), which stimulate the proliferation of vascular smooth muscle cells and their migration to the arterial intima. These cells also secrete collagenous matrix, which forms the cap of the atherosclerotic plaque.

Atherosclerotic plaque rupture. Growing plaque is a dynamic structure; the fibrous cap continues to be remodelled and during this process its component proteins are digested by proteolytic enzymes secreted by macrophages, such as collagenase. Such a highly cellular plaque may rupture, which exposes its lipid interior to the bloodstream. Because the content of the plaque core is highly thrombogenic, a wall thrombus may form quickly, block the arterial lumen and cause ischaemia, leading to tissue necrosis (a myocardial infarction or stroke).

Cardiovascular risk factors

Atherosclerosis is a metabolic disorder associated with abnormalities of both lipid and carbohydrate metabolism, the development of which is influenced by genetic factors and by environment/lifestyle. Cardiovascular risk factors such as smoking, dyslipidaemia, diabetes or hypertension are all associated with endothelial damage (Fig. 3.60.1). The so-called lipid hypothesis of atherosclerosis proposes that the amount of atherogenic particles in blood correlates with lipid deposition in the arteries. Lowering plasma LDL using lipid-lowering drugs has been shown to reduce the number of ischaemic events.

Disordered carbohydrate metabolism (glucose intolerance and diabetes mellitus) has also been linked with an increased risk of atherosclerosis. In particular, the association with hypertension and dyslipidaemia (known as the metabolic syndrome; Ch. 52) seem to increase the cardiovascular risk.

The development of atherosclerosis is also related to diet and is particularly associated with high consumption of saturated fat. Mono- and polyunsaturated fatty acids, particularly those contained in fish oil, appear to be protective. Exercise and weight reduction decrease cardiovascular risk by decreasing the incidence of the metabolic syndrome and diabetes mellitus.

GENERALIZED ATHEROSCLEROSIS

A 60-year-old man with a history of stable angina complained of pain in both calves on walking that was normally relieved by a few minutes of rest. An arteriogram demonstrated narrowing of the common femoral artery. Also, a left carotid bruit was observed. Laboratory results showed elevated total cholesterol, low HDL-cholesterol and a total cholesterol to HDL-cholesterol ratio of 7.0 (values > 5.0 are associated with high cardiovascular risk). His blood pressure was 120/80 mmHg. These are signs of generalized atherosclerosis affecting coronary arteries (angina), cerebrovascular vessels (carotid bruit) and peripheral arteries (intermittent claudication).

The management would include the medical treatment of angina and an aggressive treatment of the lipid disorder. He was considered for the angioplasty of the femoral artery.

61. Application of biochemistry to clinical practice: the work of clinical laboratories

Questions
- Which laboratory tests are commonly used to assess renal function?
- Which tests are helpful in the diagnosis of myocardial infarction?
- Which tests would you perform to assess a person's cardiovascular risk?

Biochemistry applied to clinical practice is known as clinical biochemistry. Tests performed in hospital laboratories on blood, urine and other body fluids, provide an insight into the state of metabolism and are a hugely important diagnostic tool.

Main groups of laboratory tests

The most common laboratory tests (Fig. 3.61.1) include

- **electrolyte measurements**: sodium, potassium, bicarbonate and chloride; also calcium, phosphate and magnesium
- **renal function**: urea and creatinine
- **liver function**: bilirubin and hepatic marker enzymes aspartate aminotransferase (AST), alanine aminotransferase (ALT), alkaline phosphatase and gamma-glutamyltranspeptidase (GGT)
- **plasma glucose**.
- **lipids**: total cholesterol, triacylglycerols (triglycerides), low density lipoprotein (LDL) and high density lipoprotein (HDL) are essential tools in cardiovascular prevention

- **endocrine testing** often requires complex function tests designed to stimulate or suppress the secretion of an endocrine gland
  —thyroid hormones and cortisol: most common hormones measured in clinical practice
  —gonadotrophins and gonadal steroids: important in the diagnosis of infertility
  —pituitary hormones: diagnosis and assessment of pituitary tumours
- **cardiac markers**: a major component of the diagnosis of myocardial infarction, in addition to clinical symptoms and electrocardiography; currently the principal test is the measurement of cardiac troponin (either troponin T or troponin I), which has superseded other enzymatic markers such as the MB isoenzyme of creatine kinase
- **tumour markers**: increasingly, measurement of tumour-associated molecules is used to help in the early detection of cancer
- **drugs**: laboratory tests are used to monitor plasma concentrations of prescribed drugs to optimize their dosage and avoid toxicity, particularly in antiepileptic treatment, cancer chemotherapy and treatment of cardiac failure with digoxin
- **toxicological analyses**: for poisoning and drugs of abuse.

Point-of-care testing
So-called point of care testing (POCT) provides instant measurements in intensive care units or in outpatient clinics.

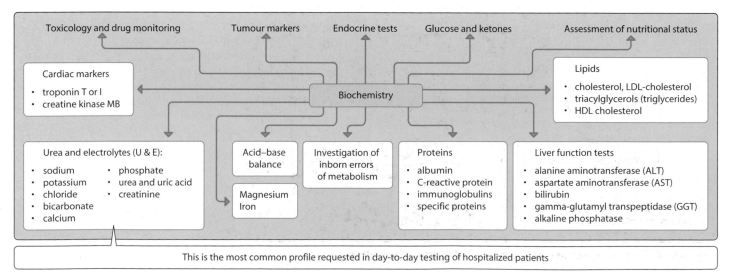

Fig. 3.61.1 The main groups of laboratory tests in clinical biochemistry.

POCT systems are most commonly used for the measurement of blood gases and plasma glucose. A variant of POCT is tests performed by patients themselves, such as glucose measurements by diabetic persons.

The clinical laboratory

The clinical laboratory in a large hospital usually performs several million tests a year. The testing is divided into three stages (Fig. 3.61.2):

  preanalytical: sample collection and transport to the laboratory
  analytical: the actual measurements and quality control
  postanalytical: data interpretation.

Considerations at the preanalytical stage include the type of sample to be taken (whole blood, plasma or serum), an appropriate preservative or anticoagulant, the timing of a sample and any required patient preparation. Many tests require simply a clotted sample of blood and the analyses are performed on the serum. When plasma is required, an anticoagulant is used to prevent clotting. A common anticoagulant is EDTA (ethylenediaminetetraacetic acid; a calcium chelator), which is particularly appropriate for blood cell counts and other haematological examinations. Sodium fluoride, an inhibitor of glycolysis, is used if glucose is to be measured. Sampling time is important; for example, the fasting glucose concentration has different reference ranges from the postprandial sample.

In a laboratory, the common tests are performed using automated analysers that handle large numbers of samples. These machines can be run in a random access mode that enables the construction of individual test profiles out of the broad test menu. Most laboratories have an emergency section that offers fast measurements of a limited range of substances.

Laboratory data are incorporated into the hospital data-processing systems; this enables results to be delivered directly to patients' records, and on-screen viewing by the ward or clinic staff.

What next? Genetics, proteomics and metabolomics

The three major areas of current research are the development of genetic testing (**genomics**) and the establishment of comprehensive protein profiles (**proteomics**) and metabolite profiles (**metabolomics**). The hope is that combining these three approaches will not only enable more precise diagnosis of many disorders but will also allow individualized profiles to be constructed, for example for drug sensitivity and response. This is known as **pharmacogenomics**. Similarly, nutritional genomics may allow the prediction of individual effects, or indeed the need for specific diets. Biochemistry and its applications to medicine continue to evolve.

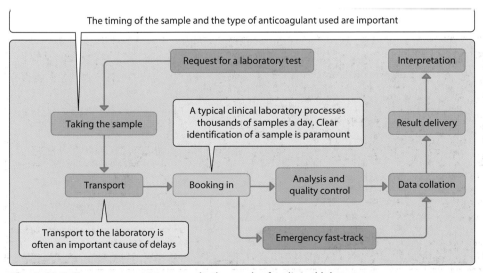

Fig. 3.61.2 From a request to a result: the work of a clinical laboratory.

62. Biochemistry-informed approach to clinical medicine

The point of learning biochemistry as a medical student is to be able to apply it in clinical situations. How could 'biochemical thinking' influence your clinical practice?

The process of diagnosis has many layers. The key points are listening to a person, keenly observing and performing clinical examination. Within this, however, considerations of metabolic status, and of many issues covered in this book, play a substantial part (Fig. 3.62.1). The list below contains the metabolism-related questions a clinician would seek an answer to at the bedside.

What is the patient's respiratory and cardiovascular status? Is the O₂ delivery adequate (the ABC of resuscitation is **airways, breathing, circulation**)? What is the haemoglobin level? Is there anaemia?

What is the water balance? Is the patient well hydrated, over-hydrated or dehydrated?

What is the electrolyte status? In particular, are there any potassium or sodium ion disturbances that need correcting? What is the renal function? Is the urine output (i.e. the excretion of metabolic products, particularly nitrogen) adequate?

What is the status of carbohydrate metabolism? Is the patient hyperglycaemic or hypoglycaemic?

What is the status of lipid transport? Are there abnormal lipoprotein concentrations?

Is the patient catabolic or anabolic?

What is the state of the gastrointestinal system? Is there an adequate digestion and absorption of nutrients? What is the liver function?

What is the nutritional status? Is there a need for nutritional support?

What tests to request? Which tests are needed to obtain answers to the above questions? Will these tests need to be carried out in a fasting state or postprandially?

There is little doubt that knowledge of biochemistry helps to provide informed answers to these questions. This is, I believe, the most important argument for learning it.

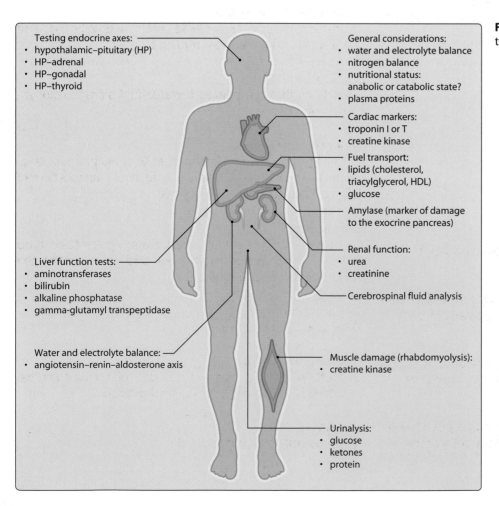

Fig. 3.62.1 Contribution of biochemistry to clinical assessment.

Testing endocrine axes:
- hypothalamic–pituitary (HP)
- HP–adrenal
- HP–gonadal
- HP–thyroid

General considerations:
- water and electrolyte balance
- nitrogen balance
- nutritional status: anabolic or catabolic state?
- plasma proteins

Cardiac markers:
- troponin I or T
- creatine kinase

Fuel transport:
- lipids (cholesterol, triacylglycerol, HDL)
- glucose

Amylase (marker of damage to the exocrine pancreas)

Renal function:
- urea
- creatinine

Cerebrospinal fluid analysis

Liver function tests:
- aminotransferases
- bilirubin
- alkaline phosphatase
- gamma-glutamyl transpeptidase

Water and electrolyte balance:
- angiotensin–renin–aldosterone axis

Muscle damage (rhabdomyolysis):
- creatine kinase

Urinalysis:
- glucose
- ketones
- protein

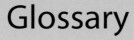

Glossary

Abbreviations

ALT	alanine transaminase
AST	aspartate transaminase
DAG	diacylglycerol
DHAP	dihydroxyacetone phosphate
DNA	deoxyribonucleic acid
F1,6BP	fructose 1,6-bisphosphate
F2,6-BP	fructose 2,6-bisphosphate
F6P	fructose 6-phosphate
FAD	flavin adenine dinucleotide
FMN	flavin adenine mononucleotide
GABA	gamma-aminobutyric acid
Glc6P	glucose 6-phosphate
HMG	hydroxymethylglutaryl
IP_3	inositol 1,4,5-triphosphate
NAD^+	nicotinamide adenine dinucleotide
NADP	nicotinamide adenine dinucleotide phosphate
PDH	pyruvate dehydrogenase
PEP	phosphoenolpyruvate
PEPCK	phosphoenolpyruvate carboxykinase
PFK	phosphofructokinase-1
PKA	protein kinase A
RNA	ribonucleic acid

Terms

Acid
A substance that dissociates into protons and a conjugate base

Acidaemia
A high hydrogen ion concentration (low blood pH)

Acidosis
A process leading to an increase in hydrogen ion concentration in the extracellular fluid (a decrease in pH)

Adenosine trisphosphate (ATP)
A nucleotide possessing high-energy bonds that serves as a vehicle for energy transfer in biological systems

Adipokines
Hormone-like molecules secreted by the adipose tissue; the most important adipokines are adiponectin and leptin

Alkalaemia
A low concentration of hydrogen ion (high blood pH)

Alkalosis
A process leading to a decrease in hydrogen ion concentration in the extracellular fluid (an increase in pH)

Allosterism
Changes in the spatial structure of multisubunit enzymes, induced by different effectors; binding of the effector leads to either activation or inhibition of the enzyme

Amphibolic reaction (or pathway)
A reaction or pathway that can be both catabolic and anabolic, e.g. the Krebs cycle

Amphipathic molecule
A molecule that possesses both hydrophobic and hydrophilic domains (e.g. phospholipids)

Anabolism
Reactions that are geared towards fuel storage, biosynthesis and growth

Anaplerotic reaction
A 'filling up', or replenishing, reaction; anaplerotic reactions feed into the Krebs cycle to avoid exhaustion of metabolites such as oxaloacetate

Apoprotein
A protein component of lipoproteins; apoproteins bind to cellular membrane receptors and thus control the metabolism of lipoproteins

Aquaporins
Membrane water channels

Asymmetric carbon
A carbon that is bonded to four different chemical residues, e.g. as in the amino acid molecule

Ataxia
An impairment of motor activity

Autocrine regulation
Regulation of cellular function by substances (such as cytokines) released by the cell itself

Basal metabolic rate (BMR)
The rate of energy utilization at rest and in the thermoneutral environment

Base
A substance that attracts protons

Body mass index (BMI)
A ratio between weight (in kilograms) and the height squared (in metres) used as a key indicator of nutritional status

Buffer
A mixture of a weak (poorly dissociated) acid and its salt; a buffer solution minimizes the changes in hydrogen ion concentration on the addition of acid or base

Catabolism
Reactions that are geared towards fuel utilization, energy-release and substance degradation

Cheilitis
The inflammation of corners of the mouth

Coenzyme
A substance (often a nucleotide, vitamin or trace metal) which participates in an enzymatic reaction by accepting and donating electrons or functional groups and is required for the reaction but differs from substrate. Coenzymes are regenerated in another reaction. In contrast to prosthetic groups, coenzymes are not structural parts of enzyme molecules

Covalent bond
A stable chemical bond based on the sharing of electrons between two atoms (common electron orbitals)

Creatine phosphate
A high-energy compound that is able to convert ADP to ATP; it is important as an 'instant energy donor' in muscle during anaerobic bursts of activity

Disaccharide
A carbohydrate molecule composed of two monosaccharides

EC number
The number assigned to an enzyme by the Enzyme Commission, which describes its class and subclass

Endergonic reaction
A reaction that requires an input of energy (there is a positive change in free energy)

Endocrine function test
A test designed to induce or suppress secretion of a hormone by stimulatory or inhibitory substances; the stimulation tests are commonly used in the diagnosis of endocrine insufficiency and the suppression tests in the diagnosis of hypersecretion

Enhancer
DNA sequence with a function similar to the promoter but which may be placed at a considerable distance from the initiation site

Enzyme
A catalytic protein that decreases the energy of activation in the chemical reaction

Exergonic reaction
A reaction that releases energy (change in free energy is negative); such reactions progress spontaneously

Feedback inhibition
The mode of regulation of metabolic pathways where the product of a pathway inhibits upstream regulatory enzymes

Flavin adenine dinucleotide (FAD)
A nucleotide involved in the electron (and proton) transfer; it is normally a prosthetic group of an enzyme

G-proteins
A superfamily of low-molecular-weight proteins that are part of the endocrine signalling cascades and are activated and deactivated by guanine nucleotides

Gene
A sequence of DNA coding for one polypeptide chain

Genome
Sum of all genes

Glycaemic control
Synonymous with diabetic control: maintaining the blood glucose concentration as close to normal as possible

Glossitis
Inflammation of the tongue

Glucogenic amino acids
Amino acids that are metabolized to the intermediates of glycolysis or Krebs cycle

Gluconeogenesis
Production of glucose from non-carbohydrate sources; main substrates for gluconeogenesis are the amino acid alanine, the lipid glycerol and the glycolytic intermediate lactate

Glucose–alanine cycle
A cyclical conversion of alanine into glucose and back that operates between muscle and liver and is an integral part of gluconeogenesis

Hormone response element
A DNA sequence that binds a transcription factor

Hydrogen bond
A weak type of interaction common in proteins and nucleic acids and also essential for interaction of water dipoles with other molecules

Hydrophilic molecule
A molecule, or part of molecule, that attracts water

Hydrophobic interactions
Weak interactions between non-polar molecules or parts of molecules; they are important for the structure of proteins and nucleic acids

Hydrophobic molecule
A molecule, or part of molecule, that repels water

Incidence
The number of new cases of a disease in a population (usually per year)

Insulin resistance (hormone resistance)
A condition where tissues or cells are poorly responsive to insulin (a hormone); insulin resistance is characterized by hyperinsulinaemia because of the compensatory secretion of insulin from pancreatic islets

Intima
The layer of the arterial wall separated from the blood by a layer of endothelial cells

Ionic interactions
Weak interactions based on attraction between negatively and positively charged residues or repulsion between residues bearing the same charge

Ionotrophic receptors
Neurotransmitter receptor that have ion channels

Isoenzymes
Different forms of an enzyme catalysing the same reaction

Ketogenic amino acids
Amino acids that are metabolized to acetyl-CoA or ketone bodies

Ketone bodies
A collective name for acetoacetate, β-hydroxybuterate and acetone

Lipogenesis
Synthesis of triacylglycerols from fatty acids and glycerol phosphate; note that this is different from the synthesis of fatty acids

Lipolysis
The hydrolysis of triacylglycerols (triglycerides); this is different from beta-oxidation of fatty acids

Metabolic shuttle
A set of reactions that bypass the lack of specific membrane transport system for a metabolite; the shuttles operate across the inner mitochondrial membrane

Metabolism
The sum of all chemical reactions in the organism

Metabolome
Sum of all metabolic intermediates

Metabotrophic receptors
Receptors for neurotransmitters that act via second messengers; these receptors often share signalling cascades with hormones

Michaelis constant (K_m)
The substrate concentration at which the enzyme achieves 50% of its maximum velocity

Monosaccharide
A simple sugar that cannot be hydrolysed into further components

Monounsaturated fatty acids
Fatty acids with one double bond in the acyl chain

Neurotransmitter
A substance involved in the transmission of signals in the central or peripheral nervous system

Neutral fats
Triacylglycerols (triglycerides): esters of glycerol and fatty acids

Nicotinamide adenine dinucleotide (NAD^+)
A nucleotide involved (as coenzyme) in electron (and proton) transfer reactions

Nicotinamide adenine dinucleotide phosphate ($NADP^+$)
A nucleotide involved (as coenzyme) in electron (and proton transfer), particularly in cytoplasmic biosynthetic reactions

Nucleoside
A molecule comprising a purine or pyrimidine base and a sugar (ribose and deoxyribose)

Nucleotide
A molecule comprising a purine or pyrimidine base, a sugar (ribose and deoxyribose) and phosphate groups

Ophthalmoplegia
Paralysis of ocular muscles

Oxidative deamination
A reaction that combines oxidation with the incorporation of the amino group (e.g. that catalysed by glutamate dehydrogenase)

Oxidative phosphorylation
A process carried out by the mitochondrial respiratory chain, which combines the oxidation of NADH or $FADH_2$ with the generation of ATP

Oxidative stress
A condition where the production of reactive oxygen species (ROS) exceeds the body's capacity for their removal

pH
Negative logarithm of hydrogen ion concentration

Paracrine function
Regulation of biochemical processes by substances released locally that affect groups of cells

Peptide bond
A covalent bond linking the carboxyl group of one amino acid with the amino group of another; it is the key bond in the primary structure of proteins

Polydipsia
Drinking large amounts of fluid

Polysaccharide
A monosaccharide polymer

Polyuria
Frequent urination

Polyunsaturated fatty acids
Fatty acids with multiple double bonds in their acyl chain

Porphyrias
Rare diseases caused by enzyme deficiencies in the pathway of haem biosynthesis

Postprandial
After a meal

Post-translational modification
Modification of a protein, such as the addition of carbo-hydrate residues, that occurs after the synthesis of the polypeptide chain

Prevalence (of a disease)
The proportion of those in the base population that have the disease; usually expressed as percentage

Promoter
A DNA sequence that directs RNA polymerase to the site of transcription initiation; the promoter is usually placed within 200 base pairs from the initiation site

Prostetic group
A chemical group that is part of the enzyme molecule and participates in an enzymatic reaction

Proteome
Sum of all the proteins in the body

Reactive oxygen species (ROS)
Extremely short-lived oxygen free radicals (partially oxidized oxygen atoms), such as superoxide, which are chemically very active

Redox pair
A pair of compounds involved in the oxidation–reduction (electron transfer) reaction

Redox potential
The tendency for a compound to donate electrons

Ribozyme
Enzymatic activity associated with ribonucleic acid rather than a protein

Salvage pathways
Pathways that allow reutilization of partially degraded compounds; such pathways are important in purine and pyrimidine metabolism, where nitrogenous bases released during degradation of nucleic acids are reutilized, decreasing the need for de novo synthesis

Saturated fatty acids
Fatty acids with no double bonds in their acyl chain

Semiconservative replication of DNA
A mode of DNA replication that preserves one of the two chains of the double helix during each cell division

Stereoisomers
Compounds characterized by different spatial arrangement of residues around an asymmetric atom; stereoisomerism is particularly important for amino acids and carbohydrates

Substrate-level phosphorylation
A reaction that produces ATP outside the mitochondrial respiratory chain

Third space
Body water compartment describing water contained in body cavities such as pleural space

Transcription
The replication of the nucleotide sequence in DNA as mRNA

Transcription factors
Proteins binding to promoter or enhancer sites of the genome that regulate transcription and thus gene expression

Translation
Construction of a polypeptide chain during protein synthesis in such a way that the sequence of amino acids reflects the sequence of nucleotide-based codes in the mRNA

Triacylglycerols
Glycerol esterified, almost always, with long-chain fatty acids; the glycerol moiety can bind three similar residues or three different ones; synonym is triglycerides

Triglycerides
Synonym for triacylglycerols

Uncouplers
Substances that dissociate the process of oxidation from phosphorylation (ATP generation) in the respiratory chain

van der Waals forces
Weak interactions important in proteins and nucleic acids characterized by repulsion over small distances

Zwitterion
A molecule that possesses both positively charged and negatively charged residues at the physiological pH

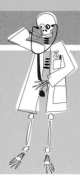

Index